20 YEARS YOUNGER
DAILY JOURNAL

20 YEARS YOUNGER

DAILY JOURNAL

Your Day-by-Day Companion

BOB GREENE

LITTLE, BROWN AND COMPANY

NEW YORK BOSTON LONDON

Little, Brown and Company
Hachette Book Group
237 Park Avenue, New York, NY 10017
www.hachettebookgroup.com

First Edition: April 2011

Little, Brown and Company is a division of Hachette Book Group, Inc. The Little, Brown name and logo are trademarks of Hachette Book Group, Inc.

The publisher is not responsible for websites (or their content) that are not owned by the publisher.

Library of Congress Cataloging-in-Publication Data

Greene, Bob (Bob W.)
    20 years younger daily journal : your day-by-day companion / Bob Greene. — 1st ed.
    p. cm.
    Summary: A companion to 20 Years Younger: look younger, feel younger, be younger! by Bob Greene; with Harold A. Lancer, Ronald L. Kotler, Diane L. McKay.
    ISBN 978-0-316-18512-7 (pbk.)
    1. Physical fitness.   2. Exercise.   3. Health.   I. Title.   II. Title: Twenty years younger daily journal.
    RA781.G7995 2011
    613.7'1—dc22

                                                                      2011000587

10 9 8 7 6 5 4 3 2 1

RRD-C

Printed in the United States of America

None are so old as those who have outlived enthusiasm.
— HENRY DAVID THOREAU

Introduction

You might think of aging as an inevitable process, but it's very possible to look, feel, and in many ways actually *be* younger than your chronological age. Accomplishing this takes some effort and discipline, but the rewards — in particular a longer, healthier, happier life — are more than worth it. The key to turning back the clock is to focus on the four pillars of anti-aging as discussed in *20 Years Younger:* exercise, nutrition, skin care, and sleep.

This journal is the companion to *20 Years Younger,* and it will help you track your progress in these four important areas. It offers a practical, manageable way to bring the book's recommendations to life. It helps you get started and stick to the program over the long term. It's also a place to set goals, track your progress, and — always a great motivator — hold yourself accountable. It is also a convenient, permanent record of your personal journey.

I've seen how adopting a healthy lifestyle with a focus on these four pillars can make people look and feel dramatically younger. And it can be a lot of fun, too! Taking a walk with a friend or hiking in a beautiful setting with your family can bring you a lot of joy, as can going to a farmers' market and tasting stellar tomatoes or sitting down to a delicious, healthy dinner. Ultimately, I hope this journal will be a useful tool as you transform yourself into a healthier person who's able to age gracefully while still maintaining a sense of youthfulness for years to come.

TRACKING PHYSICAL ACTIVITY

To combat the age-related slowdown in metabolic rate and muscle loss, and to stave off chronic diseases, you need to work your body from every angle. That's why on each of the three 20 Years Younger exercise levels outlined in the charts below, you'll be doing cardiovascular exercise, strength training, stretches, and core exercises (which strengthen the abdomen and back). It's also important to have a recreational activity that you enjoy — such as bowling or tennis. (There's a complete list of activities in *20 Years Younger* and on the website www.20yearsyounger.com.)

Look at the different levels below to determine which one is appropriate for you. Note the requirements for each type of exercise (such as 200 minutes per week of cardio in Level I) and jot them down in the exercise logs on the following pages to remind yourself of your goals. After maintaining a certain level for a few months, consider moving up to the next level to reap even more anti-aging benefits, including a greater feeling of vitality. It's also a good idea to occasionally mix it up and find alternative exercises for the moves you have been doing for six months or more. This ensures that you'll be working the same muscles in different ways, which provides a greater challenge for your body.

To see illustrations of each of the following exercises as well as recommendations for alternative moves, check out *20 Years Younger*.

LEVEL I

CARDIOVASCULAR EXERCISE

Choose from the list of anti-aging cardio activities in chapter 2 of *20 Years Younger.* Your goal: 200 minutes per week, broken up as you like. Never take off two days in a row.

Alternative for beginners: 70,000 steps per week. Count steps every day; see chapter 2 for details. (Note: The option of counting steps is available only in Level I.)

STRENGTH TRAINING

Perform each of the following moves three days a week, without taking off more than two days in a row. Start with one set with 8 to 10 repetitions per set and work up to two sets by month two and three sets by month three.

1. Heel Raise
2. Shrug Roll
3. Squat
4. Chest Press
5. Biceps Curl
6. Thumbs Down

STRETCHES

Perform each stretch two to three times in a row every day.

1. Hamstring Stretch
2. Quadriceps Stretch
3. Upper Calf Stretch
4. Lower Calf Stretch
5. Middle and Lower Back Stretch

CORE EXERCISES

Perform one set of each exercise with 15 repetitions per set every day. Work up to two sets by month two.

1. Basic Crunch

2. Upper Abdominal Crunch

3. Twisting Trunk Curl Crunch

4. Alternating Arm and Leg Raises

LIFETIME RECREATIONAL ACTIVITIES

Choose from the list of suggested activities in chapter 2 of *20 Years Younger*. Perform your chosen activity once per week. If you don't choose an activity that covers both balance and hand-eye coordination, do your strength-training exercises on a balancing apparatus, such as a wobble board or BOSU balance trainer.

LEVEL II

CARDIOVASCULAR EXERCISE

Choose from the list of anti-aging cardio activities in chapter 2 of *20 Years Younger*. Your goal: 300 minutes per week, broken up as you like. Never take off two days in a row.

STRENGTH TRAINING

Perform each of the following moves three days per week, without taking off more than two days in a row. Do three sets with 8 to 10 repetitions per set.

1. Heel Raise
2. Shrug Roll
3. Squat
4. Chest Press
5. Biceps Curl
6. Thumbs Down
7. Lunge
8. One-Arm Row
9. Dumbbell Fly
10. Triceps Extension
11. Shoulder Press
12. External Rotation

STRETCHES

Perform each stretch two to three times in a row every day.

1. Hamstring Stretch
2. Quadriceps Stretch
3. Upper Calf Stretch
4. Lower Calf Stretch
5. Middle and Lower Back Stretch

CORE EXERCISES

Perform two sets of each exercise with 15 repetitions per set every day.

1. Basic Crunch

2. Upper Abdominal Crunch

3. Twisting Trunk Curl Crunch

4. Alternating Arm and Leg Raises

5. Extended Arm Crunch

6. Vertical Leg Crunch

LIFETIME RECREATIONAL ACTIVITIES

Choose from the list of suggested activities in chapter 2 of *20 Years Younger*. Perform your chosen activity a minimum of twice per week. If you don't choose an activity that covers both balance and hand-eye coordination, do your strength-training exercises on a balancing apparatus, such as a wobble board or BOSU balance trainer.

LEVEL III

CARDIOVASCULAR EXERCISE

Choose from the list of anti-aging cardio activities in chapter 2 of *20 Years Younger*. Your goal: 400 minutes per week, broken up as you like. Never take off two days in a row.

STRENGTH TRAINING

Perform each of the following moves three days a week, without taking off more than two days in a row. Do three sets with 8 to 10 repetitions per set.

1. Heel Raise
2. Shrug Roll
3. Squat
4. Chest Press
5. Biceps Curl
6. Thumbs Down
7. Lunge
8. One-Arm Row
9. Dumbbell Fly
10. Triceps Extension
11. Shoulder Press
12. External Rotation
13. Leg Extension
14. Leg Curl
15. Lateral Raise
16. Upright Row
17. Incline Chest Press
18. Frontal Raise
19. Lat Pull Down

STRETCHES

Perform each stretch two to three times in a row every day.

1. Hamstring Stretch
2. Quadriceps Stretch
3. Upper Calf Stretch
4. Lower Calf Stretch
5. Middle and Lower Back Stretch

CORE EXERCISES

Perform two sets of each exercise with 15 repetitions per set every day.

1. Basic Crunch
2. Upper Abdominal Crunch
3. Twisting Trunk Curl Crunch
4. Alternating Arm and Leg Raises
5. Extended Arm Crunch
6. Vertical Leg Crunch
7. Reverse Trunk Curl
8. Incline Sit-Up

LIFETIME RECREATIONAL ACTIVITIES

Choose from the list of suggested activities in chapter 2 of *20 Years Younger*. Perform your chosen activity a minimum of twice per week. If you don't choose an activity that covers both balance and hand-eye coordination, do your strength-training exercises on a balancing apparatus, such as a wobble board or a BOSU balance trainer.

Tracking Your Diet

There are two key elements of an age-defying diet: It must be packed with nutrition and it must be calorie-appropriate. The diet recommended in *20 Years Younger* meets both requirements. It's rich in vitamins, minerals, and phytonutrients (beneficial plant compounds) and has the right balance of carbohydrate, protein, and fat; and by offering a variety of calorie levels, the plan helps you maintain a healthy weight—a key to staying youthful. For an added health boost, the program recommends that you take a multivitamin/mineral, a fish oil supplement, and a vitamin D/calcium supplement if needed.

The journal offers a simple tool—a diet checklist—to help you create, and stick with, this longevity-enhancing diet. The checklist instantly shows you how well you're measuring up to your dietary goals, and points out which areas need work (such as if you're coming up short on vegetable servings). Ideally, you'll fill this out every day. At a minimum, fill it out four days a week (two workdays and two nonworking days).

Here's how to use it:

- First, turn to the Daily Servings According to Calorie Intake chart on the following page. Find the number of servings in each food group appropriate for your calorie level, and jot down that number in the "Ideal Number of Servings" column in your Diet Checklist.

- At each meal, mark the number of servings consumed in each group.

- In the "Treats/beverages" section, write down the number of calories of each treat food you eat (note that you shouldn't have any treats if you're on the 1,500-calorie plan). If a food doesn't have a nutrition label (for instance, if you had a cookie from a bakery), you can find the number of calories in the food lookup tool on 20YearsYounger.com. This is also the place to record any beverages containing more than 20 calories per cup (other than milk or soy milk) that you consume. This includes soda, sweet coffee drinks, sweetened iced tea, and the like.

- Track the number of servings of superfoods you eat on the chart. (For a list of these amazing foods, turn to chapter 3 of *20 Years Younger*.) Aim to eat at least one superfood from each category every day; for fish, three times a week is fine.

You don't have to match the ideal number of servings in each group every day, but do your best to stay close. For instance, it's OK if one day you eat four fruit servings instead of the recommended two on the 1,700-calories-per-day plan. Just shave off a few calories elsewhere (for example, drop a grain serving) or work out a little harder. More important than taking in the exact number of servings is eating the best foods in each food group, outlined in chapter 3 of *20 Years Younger*. If you eat these foods and adhere to the general diet rules in that chapter (such as filling half your plate with fruits or vegetables, sticking with whole grains, and so forth), you'll wind up with a nutrient-packed diet.

Daily Servings According to Calorie Intake

As explained in chapter 3 of *20 Years Younger*, it takes a little trial and error to figure out how many daily calories you need to get down to or maintain a healthy weight. The chapter gives you guidance on picking a calorie level that's right for you. Once you've chosen one, use the following chart to find out how many daily servings of various types of food you need.

Calorie Intake	1,500	1,700	2,000	2,500
Fruits	2	2	3	4
Vegetables (and herbs and spices)	5	6	7	8
Grains/legumes/starchy vegetables	5	5	6	7
Milk/yogurt (fat-free or 1%)/soy milk	2	2	2	3
High-protein foods	6	6	7	8
Nuts/nut butters/seeds	1	1	1	2
Healthy fats	5	5	6	7
Treats/beverages	none	150	200	250

What's a Serving?

FRUIT: 1 medium-size fruit (such as an orange) or ½ cup berries, grapes, or chopped fruit

VEGETABLES: 1 cup raw greens (such as spinach or lettuce) or ½ cup chopped raw or cooked vegetables

GRAINS/LEGUMES/STARCHY VEGETABLES: 1 slice 100% whole grain bread; ½ cup cooked potatoes, corn, sweet potatoes, peas, or whole grains (such as oatmeal, whole grain pasta, or bulgur wheat); ⅓ cup cooked legumes or brown rice

MILK/YOGURT/SOY MILK: 1 cup fat-free or 1% milk or calcium-and-vitamin-D-fortified soy milk; ¾ cup fat-free or 1% plain yogurt

HIGH-PROTEIN FOODS: 1 ounce fatty fish or dark-meat poultry; 1½ ounces white fish or light-meat poultry; 1½ to 3½ ounces tofu, depending on the type (60 calories; check label); 1 to 1½ ounces tempeh (60 calories; again, check label)

NUTS/NUT BUTTERS/SEEDS: ½ ounce (about 2 tablespoons) nuts/seeds or 1 tablespoon nut butter

HEALTHY FATS: 1 teaspoon oil, mayonnaise, or healthy spread (made without partially hydrogenated oil); 1 tablespoon light mayonnaise, light healthy spread, or regular salad dressing; 2 tablespoons light salad dressing; ⅛ of a Haas avocado

WATER: 8 ounces (1 cup)

TREATS/BEVERAGES: Sweets, chips, sodas, and beverages with more than 20 calories per cup, other than milk or soy milk (serving sizes vary, so check label to find the appropriate portion for your particular treat calorie limit)

A note about alcohol: If you drink, have no more than one drink per day if you're a woman; no more than two drinks per day if you're a man. For the pros and cons of alcohol, turn to chapter 3 of *20 Years Younger.* A drink is 4 ounces of wine; 12 ounces of beer; or 1½ ounces of hard liquor, such as whisky, gin, or vodka.

Tracking Skin Care

In this journal you can also track your skin care routine. That way, you can go back and see which type of regimen and product worked best for you. Ideally, you'll be following the polish-cleanse-nourish regimen in *20 Years Younger*. You can circle *Y or N* (Yes or No) for sunscreen use.

Tracking Sleep

You can record the number of hours you sleep each night and compare that to your goal (the recommended amount of sleep is 7 to 9 hours a night). On days when you've had enough sleep, you're more likely to meet your exercise goals, because you have the energy to work out. You're also more likely to meet your diet goals, since adequate sleep helps control appetite.

Tracking Your Week

Moving toward a healthier lifestyle isn't an all-or-nothing process; you'll do better some days than others. For instance, on Monday you might hit all of your exercise goals but not quite hit the mark on the diet front. More telling than your daily progress is how you do over the course of a week; that's when more reliable trends emerge. The Weekly Summary pages are the place to track your week, giving you an instant reading of those areas where you are on track and those where you need to improve. In the Notes section at the end, write in any additional information, such as a new exercise class you started, a great recipe, an episode of emotional eating, any sleep or skin care issues, your triumphs, or any other thoughts.

YOUR "BEFORE" PHOTO

Take a photograph of yourself when you begin this program and paste it below. If you need to lose weight, take a whole-body shot in a pair of snug-fitting pants or workout clothes. If you want to improve your skin, take a close-up of your face.

Place your photo here

Your "Before" Health Stats

Consult your physician before beginning this program.

WEIGHT _____ BLOOD PRESSURE: Systolic _____ Diastolic _____

TOTAL CHOLESTEROL _____ LDL _____ HDL _____ Triglycerides _____

FASTING BLOOD GLUCOSE _____ RESTING HEART RATE _____

WAIST CIRCUMFERENCE _____

OTHER MEASUREMENTS (OPTIONAL): Chest _____ Hips _____

OTHER LAB VALUES PARTICULAR TO YOUR CONDITION (e.g., A1c, vitamin D)

_____

_____

YOUR "AFTER" PHOTO

Take a photograph of yourself three months into the program. Shoot it in a similar style to the "before" photo.

Place your photo here

Your "After" Health Stats

Record updated health stats after three months in the program.

WEIGHT _____ **BLOOD PRESSURE:** Systolic _____ Diastolic _____

TOTAL CHOLESTEROL _____ LDL _____ HDL _____ Triglycerides _____

FASTING BLOOD GLUCOSE _____ **RESTING HEART RATE** _____

WAIST CIRCUMFERENCE _____

OTHER MEASUREMENTS (OPTIONAL): Chest _____ Hips _____

OTHER LAB VALUES PARTICULAR TO YOUR CONDITION (e.g., A1c, vitamin D)

_____

_____

WEEK ONE

WEEK ONE   DATE: _____

Physical Activity

20 YEARS YOUNGER EXERCISE LEVEL: I   II   III

Cardiovascular Exercise

GOAL: Minutes (or steps) per week _____ Today's minutes (or steps) _____

Strength Training

GOAL: Sets _____ Repetitions per set _____ Days per week _____

Strength-Training Exercise	Weight/Resistance	Reps	Sets
_____			
_____			
_____			
_____			
_____			
_____			

Stretches

GOAL: Stretches _____ Days per week _____

Stretch

_____   _____

_____   _____

_____

Core Exercises

GOAL: Sets _____ Repetitions per set _____ Days per week _____

Core Exercise	Reps	Sets
_____		
_____		
_____		
_____		
_____		
_____		

Additional lifetime/recreational activities? Y N

Type: _____

> *If we all did the things we are capable of,*
> *we would astound ourselves.*
> — THOMAS EDISON

DIET CHECKLIST

Type of Food	Ideal Number of Servings	Breakfast	Lunch	Dinner	Snack(s)	Total Daily Servings
Fruits						
Vegetables (and herbs and spices)						
Grains/legumes/ starchy vegetables						
Milk/yogurt (fat-free or 1%)/soy milk						
High-protein foods						
Nuts/nut butters/seeds						
Healthy fats						
Water						
Superfoods						
Treats/beverages						

Superfoods consumed today (see the list in *20 Years Younger*) _____

_____

Did you take a multivitamin/mineral or other supplement(s)? Y N

SKIN CARE

A.M. Regimen/Products _____

_____

P.M. Regimen/Products _____

_____

Did you apply sunscreen? Y N

SLEEP

GOAL: Hours per night _____

Did you meet this goal today? Y N

WEEK ONE   DATE: _____

Physical Activity

Cardiovascular Exercise

GOAL: Minutes (or steps) per week _____ Today's minutes (or steps) _____

Strength Training

GOAL: Sets _____ Repetitions per set _____ Days per week _____

Strength-Training Exercise	Weight/Resistance	Reps	Sets

Stretches

GOAL: Stretches _____ Days per week _____

Stretch

Core Exercises

GOAL: Sets _____ Repetitions per set _____ Days per week _____

Core Exercise	Reps	Sets

Additional lifetime/recreational activities? Y N

Type: _____

> *There are no riches above a sound body.*
> — ECCLESIASTES 30:16

DIET CHECKLIST

Type of Food	Ideal Number of Servings	Breakfast	Lunch	Dinner	Snack(s)	Total Daily Servings
Fruits						
Vegetables (and herbs and spices)						
Grains/legumes/ starchy vegetables						
Milk/yogurt (fat-free or 1%)/soy milk						
High-protein foods						
Nuts/nut butters/seeds						
Healthy fats						
Water						
Superfoods						
Treats/beverages						

Superfoods consumed today (see the list in *20 Years Younger*) _____

_____

Did you take a multivitamin/mineral or other supplement(s)? Y N

SKIN CARE

A.M. Regimen/Products _____

_____

P.M. Regimen/Products _____

_____

Did you apply sunscreen? Y N

SLEEP

GOAL: Hours per night _____

Did you meet this goal today? Y N

WEEK ONE   DATE:

PHYSICAL ACTIVITY

20 YEARS YOUNGER EXERCISE LEVEL: I   II   III

Cardiovascular Exercise

GOAL: Minutes (or steps) per week _____ Today's minutes (or steps) _____

Strength Training

GOAL: Sets _____ Repetitions per set _____ Days per week _____

Strength-Training Exercise	Weight/Resistance	Reps	Sets
_____			
_____			
_____			
_____			
_____			

Stretches

GOAL: Stretches _____ Days per week _____

Stretch	
_____	_____
_____	_____
_____	

Core Exercises

GOAL: Sets _____ Repetitions per set _____ Days per week _____

Core Exercise	Reps	Sets
_____		
_____		
_____		
_____		
_____		

Additional lifetime/recreational activities? **Y N**

Type: _____

> *Energy and persistence conquer all things.*
> — BENJAMIN FRANKLIN

DIET CHECKLIST

Type of Food	Ideal Number of Servings	Breakfast	Lunch	Dinner	Snack(s)	Total Daily Servings
Fruits						
Vegetables (and herbs and spices)						
Grains/legumes/ starchy vegetables						
Milk/yogurt (fat-free or 1%)/soy milk						
High-protein foods						
Nuts/nut butters/seeds						
Healthy fats						
Water						
Superfoods						
Treats/beverages						

Superfoods consumed today (see the list in *20 Years Younger*) _____

_____

Did you take a multivitamin/mineral or other supplement(s)? Y N

SKIN CARE

A.M. Regimen/Products _____

_____

P.M. Regimen/Products _____

_____

Did you apply sunscreen? Y N

SLEEP

GOAL: Hours per night _____

Did you meet this goal today? Y N

WEEK ONE   DATE:

PHYSICAL ACTIVITY

20 YEARS YOUNGER EXERCISE LEVEL: I   II   III

Cardiovascular Exercise

GOAL: Minutes (or steps) per week _____ Today's minutes (or steps) _____

Strength Training

GOAL: Sets _____ Repetitions per set _____ Days per week _____

Strength-Training Exercise	Weight/Resistance	Reps	Sets
_____			
_____			
_____			
_____			
_____			

Stretches

GOAL: Stretches _____ Days per week _____

Stretch	
_____	_____
_____	_____
_____	

Core Exercises

GOAL: Sets _____ Repetitions per set _____ Days per week _____

Core Exercise	Reps	Sets
_____		
_____		
_____		
_____		
_____		
_____		

Additional lifetime/recreational activities? Y N

Type: _____

> *Living longer is important, but the ultimate goal is to live* well *into your later years.*
>
> — BOB GREENE

DIET CHECKLIST

Type of Food	Ideal Number of Servings	Breakfast	Lunch	Dinner	Snack(s)	Total Daily Servings
Fruits						
Vegetables (and herbs and spices)						
Grains/legumes/ starchy vegetables						
Milk/yogurt (fat-free or 1%)/soy milk						
High-protein foods						
Nuts/nut butters/seeds						
Healthy fats						
Water						
Superfoods						
Treats/beverages						

Superfoods consumed today (see the list in *20 Years Younger*) _____

_____

Did you take a multivitamin/mineral or other supplement(s)? Y N

SKIN CARE

A.M. Regimen/Products _____

_____

P.M. Regimen/Products _____

_____

Did you apply sunscreen? Y N

SLEEP

GOAL: Hours per night _____

Did you meet this goal today? Y N

WEEK ONE DATE:

PHYSICAL ACTIVITY

20 YEARS YOUNGER EXERCISE LEVEL: I II III

Cardiovascular Exercise

GOAL: Minutes (or steps) per week _____ Today's minutes (or steps) _____

Strength Training

GOAL: Sets _____ Repetitions per set _____ Days per week _____

Strength-Training Exercise	Weight/Resistance	Reps	Sets

Stretches

GOAL: Stretches _____ Days per week _____

Stretch

_____   _____

_____   _____

_____

Core Exercises

GOAL: Sets _____ Repetitions per set _____ Days per week _____

Core Exercise	Reps	Sets

Additional lifetime/recreational activities? Y N

Type: _____

> *There is only one journey, going inside yourself.*
> — RAINER MARIA RILKE

DIET CHECKLIST

Type of Food	Ideal Number of Servings	Breakfast	Lunch	Dinner	Snack(s)	Total Daily Servings
Fruits						
Vegetables (and herbs and spices)						
Grains/legumes/ starchy vegetables						
Milk/yogurt (fat-free or 1%)/soy milk						
High-protein foods						
Nuts/nut butters/seeds						
Healthy fats						
Water						
Superfoods						
Treats/beverages						

Superfoods consumed today (see the list in *20 Years Younger*) _____

_____

Did you take a multivitamin/mineral or other supplement(s)? Y N

SKIN CARE

A.M. Regimen/Products _____

_____

P.M. Regimen/Products _____

_____

Did you apply sunscreen? Y N

SLEEP

GOAL: Hours per night _____

Did you meet this goal today? Y N

Physical Activity

20 YEARS YOUNGER EXERCISE LEVEL: I   II   III

Cardiovascular Exercise

GOAL: Minutes (or steps) per week _____ Today's minutes (or steps) _____

Strength Training

GOAL: Sets _____ Repetitions per set _____ Days per week _____

Strength-Training Exercise	Weight/Resistance	Reps	Sets
_____			
_____			
_____			
_____			
_____			
_____			

Stretches

GOAL: Stretches _____ Days per week _____

Stretch

_____   _____

_____   _____

_____

Core Exercises

GOAL: Sets _____ Repetitions per set _____ Days per week _____

Core Exercise	Reps	Sets
_____		
_____		
_____		
_____		
_____		

Additional lifetime/recreational activities? Y N

Type: _____

> *You can't help getting older, but you don't have to get old.*
> — George Burns

Diet Checklist

Type of Food	Ideal Number of Servings	Breakfast	Lunch	Dinner	Snack(s)	Total Daily Servings
Fruits						
Vegetables (and herbs and spices)						
Grains/legumes/ starchy vegetables						
Milk/yogurt (fat-free or 1%)/soy milk						
High-protein foods						
Nuts/nut butters/seeds						
Healthy fats						
Water						
Superfoods						
Treats/beverages						

Superfoods consumed today (see the list in *20 Years Younger*) _____
_____

Did you take a multivitamin/mineral or other supplement(s)? Y N

Skin Care

A.M. Regimen/Products _____

_____

P.M. Regimen/Products _____

_____

Did you apply sunscreen? Y N

Sleep

GOAL: Hours per night _____

Did you meet this goal today? Y N

WEEK ONE   DATE:

Physical Activity

20 YEARS YOUNGER EXERCISE LEVEL: I   II   III

Cardiovascular Exercise

GOAL: Minutes (or steps) per week _____ Today's minutes (or steps) _____

Strength Training

GOAL: Sets _____ Repetitions per set _____ Days per week _____

Strength-Training Exercise	Weight/Resistance	Reps	Sets
_____			
_____			
_____			
_____			
_____			
_____			

Stretches

GOAL: Stretches _____ Days per week _____

Stretch

_____   _____

_____   _____

_____

Core Exercises

GOAL: Sets _____ Repetitions per set _____ Days per week _____

Core Exercise	Reps	Sets
_____		
_____		
_____		
_____		
_____		
_____		

Additional lifetime/recreational activities? Y N

Type: _____

> *Each day do something that will inch you towards a better tomorrow.*
>
> — DOUG FIREBAUGH

DIET CHECKLIST

Type of Food	Ideal Number of Servings	Breakfast	Lunch	Dinner	Snack(s)	Total Daily Servings
Fruits						
Vegetables (and herbs and spices)						
Grains/legumes/ starchy vegetables						
Milk/yogurt (fat-free or 1%)/soy milk						
High-protein foods						
Nuts/nut butters/seeds						
Healthy fats						
Water						
Superfoods						
Treats/beverages						

Superfoods consumed today (see the list in *20 Years Younger*) _____
_____

Did you take a multivitamin/mineral or other supplement(s)? Y N

SKIN CARE

A.M. Regimen/Products _____
_____

P.M. Regimen/Products _____
_____

Did you apply sunscreen? Y N

SLEEP

GOAL: Hours per night _____

Did you meet this goal today? Y N

WEEKLY SUMMARY

WEEK ONE   DATE: _____

20 YEARS YOUNGER EXERCISE LEVEL: I   II   III

PHYSICAL ACTIVITY

Cardiovascular Exercise

GOAL: Minutes (or steps) per week _____

Did you meet or exceed this goal? Y N

Strength Training

GOAL: Number of exercises _____ Sets _____

　　　　　Repetitions per set _____ Days per week _____

Did you meet or exceed this goal? Y N

Stretches

GOAL: Stretches _____ Days per week _____

Did you meet or exceed this goal? Y N

Core Exercises

GOAL: Exercises _____ Sets _____

　　　　　Repetitions per set _____ Days per week _____

Did you meet or exceed this goal? Y N

Lifetime/Recreational Activities

GOAL: Time(s) per week _____

Did you meet or exceed this goal? Y N

DIET

GOAL: Eat the ideal number of servings from each food group —
　　　　　or get very close — at least five days a week

Did you meet or exceed this goal? Y N

GOAL: Eat at least one superfood from each food group daily

Did you meet or exceed this goal? Y N

GOAL: Take a multivitamin/mineral or other supplement(s) daily

Did you meet this goal? Y N

Skin Care

GOAL: Perform skin care regimen daily in the a.m. and p.m.

Did you meet this goal? Y N

GOAL: Apply sunscreen when needed

Did you meet this goal? Y N

Sleep

GOAL: Hours per night _____

Did you meet this goal? Y N

Notes

_____
_____
_____
_____
_____
_____
_____
_____
_____
_____
_____
_____
_____
_____
_____
_____
_____
_____
_____
_____
_____
_____
_____
_____
_____
_____

WEEK TWO

WEEK TWO   DATE:

_____

PHYSICAL ACTIVITY

20 YEARS YOUNGER EXERCISE LEVEL: I   II   III

Cardiovascular Exercise

GOAL: Minutes (or steps) per week _____ Today's minutes (or steps) _____

Strength Training

GOAL: Sets _____ Repetitions per set _____ Days per week _____

Strength-Training Exercise	Weight/Resistance	Reps	Sets
_____			
_____			
_____			
_____			
_____			

Stretches

GOAL: Stretches _____ Days per week _____

Stretch

_____   _____

_____   _____

_____

Core Exercises

GOAL: Sets _____ Repetitions per set _____ Days per week _____

Core Exercise	Reps	Sets
_____		
_____		
_____		
_____		
_____		

Additional lifetime/recreational activities? **Y N**

Type: _____

> *Today a new sun rises for me; everything lives, everything is animated, everything seems to speak to me of passion, everything invites me to cherish it.*
>
> — ANNE DE L'ENCLOS

DIET CHECKLIST

Type of Food	Ideal Number of Servings	Breakfast	Lunch	Dinner	Snack(s)	Total Daily Servings
Fruits						
Vegetables (and herbs and spices)						
Grains/legumes/ starchy vegetables						
Milk/yogurt (fat-free or 1%)/soy milk						
High-protein foods						
Nuts/nut butters/seeds						
Healthy fats						
Water						
Superfoods						
Treats/beverages						

Superfoods consumed today (see the list in *20 Years Younger*) _____

_____

Did you take a multivitamin/mineral or other supplement(s)? Y N

SKIN CARE

A.M. Regimen/Products _____

_____

P.M. Regimen/Products _____

_____

Did you apply sunscreen? Y N

SLEEP

GOAL: Hours per night _____

Did you meet this goal today? Y N

WEEK TWO DATE: _____

PHYSICAL ACTIVITY

20 YEARS YOUNGER EXERCISE LEVEL: I   II   III

Cardiovascular Exercise

GOAL: Minutes (or steps) per week _____ Today's minutes (or steps) _____

Strength Training

GOAL: Sets _____ Repetitions per set _____ Days per week _____

Strength-Training Exercise	Weight/Resistance	Reps	Sets

Stretches

GOAL: Stretches _____ Days per week _____

Stretch

_____   _____

_____   _____

_____

Core Exercises

GOAL: Sets _____ Repetitions per set _____ Days per week _____

Core Exercise	Reps	Sets

Additional lifetime/recreational activities? Y N

Type: _____

> *We are what we repeatedly do. Excellence,*
> *therefore, is not an act but a habit.*
> — ARISTOTLE

DIET CHECKLIST

Type of Food	Ideal Number of Servings	Breakfast	Lunch	Dinner	Snack(s)	Total Daily Servings
Fruits						
Vegetables (and herbs and spices)						
Grains/legumes/ starchy vegetables						
Milk/yogurt (fat-free or 1%)/soy milk						
High-protein foods						
Nuts/nut butters/seeds						
Healthy fats						
Water						
Superfoods						
Treats/beverages						

Superfoods consumed today (see the list in *20 Years Younger*) _____

_____

Did you take a multivitamin/mineral or other supplement(s)? Y N

SKIN CARE

A.M. Regimen/Products _____

_____

P.M. Regimen/Products _____

_____

Did you apply sunscreen? Y N

SLEEP

GOAL: Hours per night _____

Did you meet this goal today? Y N

WEEK TWO   DATE: _____

PHYSICAL ACTIVITY

20 YEARS YOUNGER EXERCISE LEVEL: I   II   III

Cardiovascular Exercise

GOAL: Minutes (or steps) per week _____ Today's minutes (or steps) _____

Strength Training

GOAL: Sets _____ Repetitions per set _____ Days per week _____

Strength-Training Exercise	Weight/Resistance	Reps	Sets
_____			
_____			
_____			
_____			
_____			
_____			

Stretches

GOAL: Stretches _____ Days per week _____

Stretch	
_____	_____
_____	_____
_____	

Core Exercises

GOAL: Sets _____ Repetitions per set _____ Days per week _____

Core Exercise	Reps	Sets
_____		
_____		
_____		
_____		
_____		
_____		

Additional lifetime/recreational activities? **Y N**

Type: _____

> *You can't be complacent if you want to age gracefully.*
> — BOB GREENE

DIET CHECKLIST

Type of Food	Ideal Number of Servings	Breakfast	Lunch	Dinner	Snack(s)	Total Daily Servings
Fruits						
Vegetables (and herbs and spices)						
Grains/legumes/ starchy vegetables						
Milk/yogurt (fat-free or 1%)/soy milk						
High-protein foods						
Nuts/nut butters/seeds						
Healthy fats						
Water						
Superfoods						
Treats/beverages						

Superfoods consumed today (see the list in *20 Years Younger*) _____

_____

Did you take a multivitamin/mineral or other supplement(s)? Y N

SKIN CARE

A.M. Regimen/Products _____

_____

P.M. Regimen/Products _____

_____

Did you apply sunscreen? Y N

SLEEP

GOAL: Hours per night _____

Did you meet this goal today? Y N

WEEK TWO

DATE: _____

PHYSICAL ACTIVITY

20 YEARS YOUNGER EXERCISE LEVEL: I   II   III

Cardiovascular Exercise

GOAL: Minutes (or steps) per week _____ Today's minutes (or steps) _____

Strength Training

GOAL: Sets _____ Repetitions per set _____ Days per week _____

Strength-Training Exercise	Weight/Resistance	Reps	Sets

Stretches

GOAL: Stretches _____ Days per week _____

Stretch	

Core Exercises

GOAL: Sets _____ Repetitions per set _____ Days per week _____

Core Exercise	Reps	Sets

Additional lifetime/recreational activities? Y N

Type: _____

> *The longer I live, the more beautiful life becomes.*
> — FRANK LLOYD WRIGHT

DIET CHECKLIST

Type of Food	Ideal Number of Servings	Breakfast	Lunch	Dinner	Snack(s)	Total Daily Servings
Fruits						
Vegetables (and herbs and spices)						
Grains/legumes/ starchy vegetables						
Milk/yogurt (fat-free or 1%)/soy milk						
High-protein foods						
Nuts/nut butters/seeds						
Healthy fats						
Water						
Superfoods						
Treats/beverages						

Superfoods consumed today (see the list in *20 Years Younger*) _____

_____

Did you take a multivitamin/mineral or other supplement(s)? Y N

SKIN CARE

A.M. Regimen/Products _____

_____

P.M. Regimen/Products _____

_____

Did you apply sunscreen? Y N

SLEEP

GOAL: Hours per night _____

Did you meet this goal today? Y N

WEEK TWO   DATE: _____

PHYSICAL ACTIVITY

20 YEARS YOUNGER EXERCISE LEVEL: I   II   III

Cardiovascular Exercise

GOAL: Minutes (or steps) per week _____ Today's minutes (or steps) _____

Strength Training

GOAL: Sets _____ Repetitions per set _____ Days per week _____

Strength-Training Exercise	Weight/Resistance	Reps	Sets

Stretches

GOAL: Stretches _____ Days per week _____

Stretch

_____   _____

_____   _____

_____

Core Exercises

GOAL: Sets _____ Repetitions per set _____ Days per week _____

Core Exercise	Reps	Sets

Additional lifetime/recreational activities? Y N

Type: _____

> *Success is the sum of small efforts,*
> *repeated day in and day out.*
> — ROBERT COLLIER

DIET CHECKLIST

Type of Food	Ideal Number of Servings	Breakfast	Lunch	Dinner	Snack(s)	Total Daily Servings
Fruits						
Vegetables (and herbs and spices)						
Grains/legumes/ starchy vegetables						
Milk/yogurt (fat-free or 1%)/soy milk						
High-protein foods						
Nuts/nut butters/seeds						
Healthy fats						
Water						
Superfoods						
Treats/beverages						

Superfoods consumed today (see the list in *20 Years Younger*) _____

_____

Did you take a multivitamin/mineral or other supplement(s)? Y N

SKIN CARE

A.M. Regimen/Products _____

_____

P.M. Regimen/Products _____

_____

Did you apply sunscreen? Y N

SLEEP

GOAL: Hours per night _____

Did you meet this goal today? Y N

WEEK TWO   DATE:

Physical Activity

20 YEARS YOUNGER EXERCISE LEVEL: I   II   III

Cardiovascular Exercise

GOAL: Minutes (or steps) per week _____ Today's minutes (or steps) _____

Strength Training

GOAL: Sets _____ Repetitions per set _____ Days per week _____

Strength-Training Exercise	Weight/Resistance	Reps	Sets

Stretches

GOAL: Stretches _____ Days per week _____

Stretch	
_____	_____
_____	_____
_____	

Core Exercises

GOAL: Sets _____ Repetitions per set _____ Days per week _____

Core Exercise	Reps	Sets

Additional lifetime/recreational activities? **Y N**

Type: _____

> *None are so old as those who have outlived enthusiasm.*
> — HENRY DAVID THOREAU

DIET CHECKLIST

Type of Food	Ideal Number of Servings	Breakfast	Lunch	Dinner	Snack(s)	Total Daily Servings
Fruits						
Vegetables (and herbs and spices)						
Grains/legumes/ starchy vegetables						
Milk/yogurt (fat-free or 1%)/soy milk						
High-protein foods						
Nuts/nut butters/seeds						
Healthy fats						
Water						
Superfoods						
Treats/beverages						

Superfoods consumed today (see the list in *20 Years Younger*) _____
_____

Did you take a multivitamin/mineral or other supplement(s)? Y N

SKIN CARE

A.M. Regimen/Products _____
_____

P.M. Regimen/Products _____
_____

Did you apply sunscreen? Y N

SLEEP

GOAL: Hours per night _____

Did you meet this goal today? Y N

WEEK TWO   DATE:

Physical Activity

20 YEARS YOUNGER EXERCISE LEVEL: I   II   III

Cardiovascular Exercise

GOAL: Minutes (or steps) per week _____ Today's minutes (or steps) _____

Strength Training

GOAL: Sets _____ Repetitions per set _____ Days per week _____

Strength-Training Exercise	Weight/Resistance	Reps	Sets

Stretches

GOAL: Stretches _____ Days per week _____

Stretch

_____   _____

_____   _____

_____

Core Exercises

GOAL: Sets _____ Repetitions per set _____ Days per week _____

Core Exercise	Reps	Sets

Additional lifetime/recreational activities? Y N

Type: _____

DIET CHECKLIST

Type of Food	Ideal Number of Servings	Breakfast	Lunch	Dinner	Snack(s)	Total Daily Servings
Fruits						
Vegetables (and herbs and spices)						
Grains/legumes/ starchy vegetables						
Milk/yogurt (fat-free or 1%)/soy milk						
High-protein foods						
Nuts/nut butters/seeds						
Healthy fats						
Water						
Superfoods						
Treats/beverages						

Superfoods consumed today (see the list in *20 Years Younger*) _____
_____

Did you take a multivitamin/mineral or other supplement(s)? Y N

SKIN CARE

A.M. Regimen/Products _____

_____

P.M. Regimen/Products _____

_____

Did you apply sunscreen? Y N

SLEEP

GOAL: Hours per night _____

Did you meet this goal today? Y N

WEEKLY SUMMARY

WEEK TWO   DATE:

20 YEARS YOUNGER EXERCISE LEVEL: I   II   III

PHYSICAL ACTIVITY

Cardiovascular Exercise

GOAL: Minutes (or steps) per week _____

Did you meet or exceed this goal? **Y N**

Strength Training

GOAL: Number of exercises _____ Sets _____

Repetitions per set _____ Days per week _____

Did you meet or exceed this goal? **Y N**

Stretches

GOAL: Stretches _____ Days per week _____

Did you meet or exceed this goal? **Y N**

Core Exercises

GOAL: Exercises _____ Sets _____

Repetitions per set _____ Days per week _____

Did you meet or exceed this goal? **Y N**

Lifetime/Recreational Activities

GOAL: Time(s) per week _____

Did you meet or exceed this goal? **Y N**

DIET

GOAL: Eat the ideal number of servings from each food group—
or get very close—at least five days a week

Did you meet or exceed this goal? **Y N**

GOAL: Eat at least one superfood from each food group daily

Did you meet or exceed this goal? **Y N**

GOAL: Take a multivitamin/mineral or other supplement(s) daily

Did you meet this goal? Y N

Skin Care

GOAL: Perform skin care regimen daily in the a.m. and p.m.

Did you meet this goal? Y N

GOAL: Apply sunscreen when needed

Did you meet this goal? Y N

Sleep

GOAL: Hours per night _____

Did you meet this goal? Y N

Notes

_____
_____
_____
_____
_____
_____
_____
_____
_____
_____
_____
_____
_____
_____
_____
_____
_____
_____
_____
_____
_____
_____
_____
_____

WEEK THREE

WEEK THREE   DATE:

PHYSICAL ACTIVITY

20 YEARS YOUNGER EXERCISE LEVEL: I   II   III

Cardiovascular Exercise

GOAL: Minutes (or steps) per week _____ Today's minutes (or steps) _____

Strength Training

GOAL: Sets _____ Repetitions per set _____ Days per week _____

Strength-Training Exercise	Weight/Resistance	Reps	Sets

Stretches

GOAL: Stretches _____ Days per week _____

Stretch	

Core Exercises

GOAL: Sets _____ Repetitions per set _____ Days per week _____

Core Exercise	Reps	Sets

Additional lifetime/recreational activities? Y N

Type: _____

*The life you lead and the decisions you make every day
are largely responsible for how quickly, profoundly,
and noticeably you age.*

— BOB GREENE

DIET CHECKLIST

Type of Food	Ideal Number of Servings	Breakfast	Lunch	Dinner	Snack(s)	Total Daily Servings
Fruits						
Vegetables (and herbs and spices)						
Grains/legumes/ starchy vegetables						
Milk/yogurt (fat-free or 1%)/soy milk						
High-protein foods						
Nuts/nut butters/seeds						
Healthy fats						
Water						
Superfoods						
Treats/beverages						

Superfoods consumed today (see the list in *20 Years Younger*) _____

_____

Did you take a multivitamin/mineral or other supplement(s)? Y N

SKIN CARE

A.M. Regimen/Products _____

_____

P.M. Regimen/Products _____

_____

Did you apply sunscreen? Y N

SLEEP

GOAL: Hours per night _____

Did you meet this goal today? Y N

WEEK THREE   DATE:

Physical Activity

20 YEARS YOUNGER EXERCISE LEVEL: I   II   III

Cardiovascular Exercise

GOAL: Minutes (or steps) per week _____ Today's minutes (or steps) _____

Strength Training

GOAL: Sets _____ Repetitions per set _____ Days per week _____

Strength-Training Exercise	Weight/Resistance	Reps	Sets

Stretches

GOAL: Stretches _____ Days per week _____

Stretch

_____   _____

_____   _____

_____

Core Exercises

GOAL: Sets _____ Repetitions per set _____ Days per week _____

Core Exercise	Reps	Sets

Additional lifetime/recreational activities? Y N

Type: _____

> *Renew thyself completely each day; do it again,
> and again, and forever again.*
>
> — CHINESE INSCRIPTION CITED BY THOREAU IN *WALDEN*

DIET CHECKLIST

Type of Food	Ideal Number of Servings	Breakfast	Lunch	Dinner	Snack(s)	Total Daily Servings
Fruits						
Vegetables (and herbs and spices)						
Grains/legumes/ starchy vegetables						
Milk/yogurt (fat-free or 1%)/soy milk						
High-protein foods						
Nuts/nut butters/seeds						
Healthy fats						
Water						
Superfoods						
Treats/beverages						

Superfoods consumed today (see the list in *20 Years Younger*) _____

_____

Did you take a multivitamin/mineral or other supplement(s)? Y N

SKIN CARE

A.M. Regimen/Products _____

_____

P.M. Regimen/Products _____

_____

Did you apply sunscreen? Y N

SLEEP

GOAL: Hours per night _____

Did you meet this goal today? Y N

WEEK THREE   DATE:

Physical Activity

20 YEARS YOUNGER EXERCISE LEVEL: I   II   III

Cardiovascular Exercise

GOAL: Minutes (or steps) per week _____ Today's minutes (or steps) _____

Strength Training

GOAL: Sets _____ Repetitions per set _____ Days per week _____

Strength-Training Exercise	Weight/Resistance	Reps	Sets

Stretches

GOAL: Stretches _____ Days per week _____

Stretch

_____   _____

_____   _____

_____

Core Exercises

GOAL: Sets _____ Repetitions per set _____ Days per week _____

Core Exercise	Reps	Sets

Additional lifetime/recreational activities? **Y N**

Type: _____

DIET CHECKLIST

Type of Food	Ideal Number of Servings	Breakfast	Lunch	Dinner	Snack(s)	Total Daily Servings
Fruits						
Vegetables (and herbs and spices)						
Grains/legumes/ starchy vegetables						
Milk/yogurt (fat-free or 1%)/soy milk						
High-protein foods						
Nuts/nut butters/seeds						
Healthy fats						
Water						
Superfoods						
Treats/beverages						

Superfoods consumed today (see the list in *20 Years Younger*) _____

_____

Did you take a multivitamin/mineral or other supplement(s)? Y N

SKIN CARE

A.M. Regimen/Products _____

_____

P.M. Regimen/Products _____

_____

Did you apply sunscreen? Y N

SLEEP

GOAL: Hours per night _____

Did you meet this goal today? Y N

WEEK THREE DATE:

PHYSICAL ACTIVITY

20 YEARS YOUNGER EXERCISE LEVEL: I   II   III

Cardiovascular Exercise

GOAL: Minutes (or steps) per week _____ Today's minutes (or steps) _____

Strength Training

GOAL: Sets _____ Repetitions per set _____ Days per week _____

Strength-Training Exercise	Weight/Resistance	Reps	Sets
_____			
_____			
_____			
_____			
_____			

Stretches

GOAL: Stretches _____ Days per week _____

Stretch

_____   _____

_____   _____

_____

Core Exercises

GOAL: Sets _____ Repetitions per set _____ Days per week _____

Core Exercise	Reps	Sets
_____		
_____		
_____		
_____		
_____		
_____		

Additional lifetime/recreational activities? Y N

Type: _____

> *Health is the vital principle of bliss. And exercise of health.*
> — JAMES THOMPSON

DIET CHECKLIST

Type of Food	Ideal Number of Servings	Breakfast	Lunch	Dinner	Snack(s)	Total Daily Servings
Fruits						
Vegetables (and herbs and spices)						
Grains/legumes/ starchy vegetables						
Milk/yogurt (fat-free or 1%)/soy milk						
High-protein foods						
Nuts/nut butters/seeds						
Healthy fats						
Water						
Superfoods						
Treats/beverages						

Superfoods consumed today (see the list in *20 Years Younger*) _____

_____

Did you take a multivitamin/mineral or other supplement(s)? Y N

SKIN CARE

A.M. Regimen/Products _____

_____

P.M. Regimen/Products _____

_____

Did you apply sunscreen? Y N

SLEEP

GOAL: Hours per night _____

Did you meet this goal today? Y N

WEEK THREE   DATE: _____

PHYSICAL ACTIVITY

20 YEARS YOUNGER EXERCISE LEVEL: I   II   III

Cardiovascular Exercise

GOAL: Minutes (or steps) per week _____ Today's minutes (or steps) _____

Strength Training

GOAL: Sets _____ Repetitions per set _____ Days per week _____

Strength-Training Exercise	Weight/Resistance	Reps	Sets

Stretches

GOAL: Stretches _____ Days per week _____

Stretch	
_____	_____
_____	_____
_____	

Core Exercises

GOAL: Sets _____ Repetitions per set _____ Days per week _____

Core Exercise	Reps	Sets

Additional lifetime/recreational activities? Y N

Type: _____

> *Self-awareness, self-acceptance, and self-love*
> *are lifelong processes.*
> — Bob Greene

Diet Checklist

Type of Food	Ideal Number of Servings	Breakfast	Lunch	Dinner	Snack(s)	Total Daily Servings
Fruits						
Vegetables (and herbs and spices)						
Grains/legumes/ starchy vegetables						
Milk/yogurt (fat-free or 1%)/soy milk						
High-protein foods						
Nuts/nut butters/seeds						
Healthy fats						
Water						
Superfoods						
Treats/beverages						

Superfoods consumed today (see the list in *20 Years Younger*) _____
_____

Did you take a multivitamin/mineral or other supplement(s)? **Y N**

Skin Care

A.M. Regimen/Products _____
_____

P.M. Regimen/Products _____
_____

Did you apply sunscreen? **Y N**

Sleep

GOAL: Hours per night _____

Did you meet this goal today? **Y N**

WEEK THREE DATE:

Physical Activity

20 YEARS YOUNGER EXERCISE LEVEL: I   II   III

Cardiovascular Exercise

GOAL: Minutes (or steps) per week _____ Today's minutes (or steps) _____

Strength Training

GOAL: Sets _____ Repetitions per set _____ Days per week _____

Strength-Training Exercise	Weight/Resistance	Reps	Sets

Stretches

GOAL: Stretches _____ Days per week _____

Stretch	
_____	_____
_____	_____
_____	

Core Exercises

GOAL: Sets _____ Repetitions per set _____ Days per week _____

Core Exercise	Reps	Sets

Additional lifetime/recreational activities? Y N

Type: _____

> *True life is lived when small changes occur.*
> — LEO TOLSTOY

DIET CHECKLIST

Type of Food	Ideal Number of Servings	Breakfast	Lunch	Dinner	Snack(s)	Total Daily Servings
Fruits						
Vegetables (and herbs and spices)						
Grains/legumes/ starchy vegetables						
Milk/yogurt (fat-free or 1%)/soy milk						
High-protein foods						
Nuts/nut butters/seeds						
Healthy fats						
Water						
Superfoods						
Treats/beverages						

Superfoods consumed today (see the list in *20 Years Younger*) _____
_____

Did you take a multivitamin/mineral or other supplement(s)? Y N

SKIN CARE

A.M. Regimen/Products _____
_____

P.M. Regimen/Products _____
_____

Did you apply sunscreen? Y N

SLEEP

GOAL: Hours per night _____

Did you meet this goal today? Y N

WEEK THREE   DATE: _____

PHYSICAL ACTIVITY

20 YEARS YOUNGER EXERCISE LEVEL: I   II   III

Cardiovascular Exercise

GOAL: Minutes (or steps) per week _____ Today's minutes (or steps) _____

Strength Training

GOAL: Sets _____ Repetitions per set _____ Days per week _____

Strength-Training Exercise	Weight/Resistance	Reps	Sets

Stretches

GOAL: Stretches _____ Days per week _____

Stretch

_____   _____
_____   _____
_____

Core Exercises

GOAL: Sets _____ Repetitions per set _____ Days per week _____

Core Exercise	Reps	Sets

Additional lifetime/recreational activities? Y N

Type: _____

> *Sleep is like the air we breathe; we need it to be healthy*
> *in virtually every way as well as to be safe.*
> — RONALD KOTLER, MD

DIET CHECKLIST

Type of Food	Ideal Number of Servings	Breakfast	Lunch	Dinner	Snack(s)	Total Daily Servings
Fruits						
Vegetables (and herbs and spices)						
Grains/legumes/ starchy vegetables						
Milk/yogurt (fat-free or 1%)/soy milk						
High-protein foods						
Nuts/nut butters/seeds						
Healthy fats						
Water						
Superfoods						
Treats/beverages						

Superfoods consumed today (see the list in *20 Years Younger*) _____

_____

Did you take a multivitamin/mineral or other supplement(s)? Y N

SKIN CARE

A.M. Regimen/Products _____

_____

P.M. Regimen/Products _____

_____

Did you apply sunscreen? Y N

SLEEP

GOAL: Hours per night _____

Did you meet this goal today? Y N

WEEKLY SUMMARY

WEEK THREE

DATE:

20 YEARS YOUNGER EXERCISE LEVEL: I   II   III

PHYSICAL ACTIVITY

Cardiovascular Exercise

GOAL: Minutes (or steps) per week _____

Did you meet or exceed this goal? Y N

Strength Training

GOAL: Number of exercises _____ Sets _____

Repetitions per set _____ Days per week _____

Did you meet or exceed this goal? Y N

Stretches

GOAL: Stretches _____ Days per week _____

Did you meet or exceed this goal? Y N

Core Exercises

GOAL: Exercises _____ Sets _____

Repetitions per set _____ Days per week _____

Did you meet or exceed this goal? Y N

Lifetime/Recreational Activities

GOAL: Time(s) per week _____

Did you meet or exceed this goal? Y N

DIET

GOAL: Eat the ideal number of servings from each food group —
or get very close — at least five days a week

Did you meet or exceed this goal? Y N

GOAL: Eat at least one superfood from each food group daily

Did you meet or exceed this goal? Y N

GOAL: Take a multivitamin/mineral or other supplement(s) daily

Did you meet this goal? Y N

Skin Care

GOAL: Perform skin care regimen daily in the a.m. and p.m.

Did you meet this goal? Y N

GOAL: Apply sunscreen when needed

Did you meet this goal? Y N

Sleep

GOAL: Hours per night _____

Did you meet this goal? Y N

Notes

_____
_____
_____
_____
_____
_____
_____
_____
_____
_____
_____
_____
_____
_____
_____
_____
_____
_____
_____
_____
_____
_____
_____

WEEK FOUR

WEEK FOUR   DATE: _____

Physical Activity

20 YEARS YOUNGER EXERCISE LEVEL: I   II   III

Cardiovascular Exercise

GOAL: Minutes (or steps) per week _____ Today's minutes (or steps) _____

Strength Training

GOAL: Sets _____ Repetitions per set _____ Days per week _____

Strength-Training Exercise	Weight/Resistance	Reps	Sets

Stretches

GOAL: Stretches _____ Days per week _____

Stretch

_____   _____

_____   _____

_____

Core Exercises

GOAL: Sets _____ Repetitions per set _____ Days per week _____

Core Exercise	Reps	Sets

Additional lifetime/recreational activities?   **Y N**

Type: _____

> *What is called genius is the abundance of life and health.*
> — HENRY DAVID THOREAU

DIET CHECKLIST

Type of Food	Ideal Number of Servings	Breakfast	Lunch	Dinner	Snack(s)	Total Daily Servings
Fruits						
Vegetables (and herbs and spices)						
Grains/legumes/ starchy vegetables						
Milk/yogurt (fat-free or 1%)/soy milk						
High-protein foods						
Nuts/nut butters/seeds						
Healthy fats						
Water						
Superfoods						
Treats/beverages						

Superfoods consumed today (see the list in *20 Years Younger*) _____

_____

Did you take a multivitamin/mineral or other supplement(s)? Y N

SKIN CARE

A.M. Regimen/Products _____

_____

P.M. Regimen/Products _____

_____

Did you apply sunscreen? Y N

SLEEP

GOAL: Hours per night _____

Did you meet this goal today? Y N

WEEK FOUR DATE: _____

Physical Activity

Cardiovascular Exercise

GOAL: Minutes (or steps) per week _____ Today's minutes (or steps) _____

Strength Training

GOAL: Sets _____ Repetitions per set _____ Days per week _____

Strength-Training Exercise	Weight/Resistance	Reps	Sets
_____			
_____			
_____			
_____			
_____			
_____			

Stretches

GOAL: Stretches _____ Days per week _____

Stretch

_____   _____

_____   _____

_____

Core Exercises

GOAL: Sets _____ Repetitions per set _____ Days per week _____

Core Exercise	Reps	Sets
_____		
_____		
_____		
_____		
_____		
_____		

Additional lifetime/recreational activities? Y N

Type: _____

DIET CHECKLIST

Type of Food	Ideal Number of Servings	Breakfast	Lunch	Dinner	Snack(s)	Total Daily Servings
Fruits						
Vegetables (and herbs and spices)						
Grains/legumes/ starchy vegetables						
Milk/yogurt (fat-free or 1%)/soy milk						
High-protein foods						
Nuts/nut butters/seeds						
Healthy fats						
Water						
Superfoods						
Treats/beverages						

Superfoods consumed today (see the list in *20 Years Younger*) _____

_____

Did you take a multivitamin/mineral or other supplement(s)? Y N

SKIN CARE

A.M. Regimen/Products _____

_____

P.M. Regimen/Products _____

_____

Did you apply sunscreen? Y N

SLEEP

GOAL: Hours per night _____

Did you meet this goal today? Y N

WEEK FOUR   DATE: _____

Physical Activity

20 YEARS YOUNGER EXERCISE LEVEL: I   II   III

Cardiovascular Exercise

GOAL: Minutes (or steps) per week _____ Today's minutes (or steps) _____

Strength Training

GOAL: Sets _____ Repetitions per set _____ Days per week _____

Strength-Training Exercise	Weight/Resistance	Reps	Sets

Stretches

GOAL: Stretches _____ Days per week _____

Stretch

_____   _____

_____   _____

_____

Core Exercises

GOAL: Sets _____ Repetitions per set _____ Days per week _____

Core Exercise	Reps	Sets

Additional lifetime/recreational activities? **Y   N**

Type: _____

> *The love, friendship, and companionship of others are integral to aging gracefully.*
> — BOB GREENE

DIET CHECKLIST

Type of Food	Ideal Number of Servings	Breakfast	Lunch	Dinner	Snack(s)	Total Daily Servings
Fruits						
Vegetables (and herbs and spices)						
Grains/legumes/ starchy vegetables						
Milk/yogurt (fat-free or 1%)/soy milk						
High-protein foods						
Nuts/nut butters/seeds						
Healthy fats						
Water						
Superfoods						
Treats/beverages						

Superfoods consumed today (see the list in *20 Years Younger*) _____

_____

Did you take a multivitamin/mineral or other supplement(s)? Y N

SKIN CARE

A.M. Regimen/Products _____

_____

P.M. Regimen/Products _____

_____

Did you apply sunscreen? Y N

SLEEP

GOAL: Hours per night _____

Did you meet this goal today? Y N

WEEK FOUR   DATE: _____

Physical Activity

Cardiovascular Exercise

GOAL: Minutes (or steps) per week _____ Today's minutes (or steps) _____

Strength Training

GOAL: Sets _____ Repetitions per set _____ Days per week _____

Strength-Training Exercise	Weight/Resistance	Reps	Sets
_____			
_____			
_____			
_____			
_____			
_____			

Stretches

GOAL: Stretches _____ Days per week _____

Stretch	
_____	_____
_____	_____
_____	

Core Exercises

GOAL: Sets _____ Repetitions per set _____ Days per week _____

Core Exercise	Reps	Sets
_____		
_____		
_____		
_____		
_____		
_____		

Additional lifetime/recreational activities? **Y N**

Type: _____

DIET CHECKLIST

Type of Food	Ideal Number of Servings	Breakfast	Lunch	Dinner	Snack(s)	Total Daily Servings
Fruits						
Vegetables (and herbs and spices)						
Grains/legumes/ starchy vegetables						
Milk/yogurt (fat-free or 1%)/soy milk						
High-protein foods						
Nuts/nut butters/seeds						
Healthy fats						
Water						
Superfoods						
Treats/beverages						

Superfoods consumed today (see the list in *20 Years Younger*) _____

_____

Did you take a multivitamin/mineral or other supplement(s)? Y N

SKIN CARE

A.M. Regimen/Products _____

_____

P.M. Regimen/Products _____

_____

Did you apply sunscreen? Y N

SLEEP

GOAL: Hours per night _____

Did you meet this goal today? Y N

WEEK FOUR DATE: _____

Physical Activity

20 YEARS YOUNGER EXERCISE LEVEL: I   II   III

Cardiovascular Exercise

GOAL: Minutes (or steps) per week _____ Today's minutes (or steps) _____

Strength Training

GOAL: Sets _____ Repetitions per set _____ Days per week _____

Strength-Training Exercise	Weight/Resistance	Reps	Sets

Stretches

GOAL: Stretches _____ Days per week _____

Stretch

_____   _____

_____   _____

_____

Core Exercises

GOAL: Sets _____ Repetitions per set _____ Days per week _____

Core Exercise	Reps	Sets

Additional lifetime/recreational activities? Y N

Type: _____

> *If we had no winter, the spring would not be so pleasant;*
> *if we did not sometimes taste adversity, prosperity*
> *would not be so welcome.*
> — ANNE BRADSTREET

DIET CHECKLIST

Type of Food	Ideal Number of Servings	Breakfast	Lunch	Dinner	Snack(s)	Total Daily Servings
Fruits						
Vegetables (and herbs and spices)						
Grains/legumes/ starchy vegetables						
Milk/yogurt (fat-free or 1%)/soy milk						
High-protein foods						
Nuts/nut butters/seeds						
Healthy fats						
Water						
Superfoods						
Treats/beverages						

Superfoods consumed today (see the list in *20 Years Younger*) _____

_____

Did you take a multivitamin/mineral or other supplement(s)? **Y N**

SKIN CARE

A.M. Regimen/Products _____

_____

P.M. Regimen/Products _____

_____

Did you apply sunscreen? **Y N**

SLEEP

GOAL: Hours per night _____

Did you meet this goal today? **Y N**

WEEK FOUR   DATE: _____

Physical Activity

20 YEARS YOUNGER EXERCISE LEVEL: I   II   III

Cardiovascular Exercise

GOAL: Minutes (or steps) per week _____ Today's minutes (or steps) _____

Strength Training

GOAL: Sets _____ Repetitions per set _____ Days per week _____

Strength-Training Exercise	Weight/Resistance	Reps	Sets

Stretches

GOAL: Stretches _____ Days per week _____

Stretch

_____   _____

_____   _____

_____

Core Exercises

GOAL: Sets _____ Repetitions per set _____ Days per week _____

Core Exercise	Reps	Sets

Additional lifetime/recreational activities? **Y N**

Type: _____

> *Always be a first-rate version of yourself, instead of a second-rate version of someone else.*
>
> — JUDY GARLAND

DIET CHECKLIST

Type of Food	Ideal Number of Servings	Breakfast	Lunch	Dinner	Snack(s)	Total Daily Servings
Fruits						
Vegetables (and herbs and spices)						
Grains/legumes/ starchy vegetables						
Milk/yogurt (fat-free or 1%)/soy milk						
High-protein foods						
Nuts/nut butters/seeds						
Healthy fats						
Water						
Superfoods						
Treats/beverages						

Superfoods consumed today (see the list in *20 Years Younger*) _____

_____

Did you take a multivitamin/mineral or other supplement(s)? **Y N**

SKIN CARE

A.M. Regimen/Products _____

_____

P.M. Regimen/Products _____

_____

Did you apply sunscreen? **Y N**

SLEEP

GOAL: Hours per night _____

Did you meet this goal today? **Y N**

WEEK FOUR DATE: _____

PHYSICAL ACTIVITY

20 YEARS YOUNGER EXERCISE LEVEL: I   II   III

Cardiovascular Exercise

GOAL: Minutes (or steps) per week _____ Today's minutes (or steps) _____

Strength Training

GOAL: Sets _____ Repetitions per set _____ Days per week _____

Strength-Training Exercise	Weight/Resistance	Reps	Sets

Stretches

GOAL: Stretches _____ Days per week _____

Stretch

_____   _____

_____   _____

_____

Core Exercises

GOAL: Sets _____ Repetitions per set _____ Days per week _____

Core Exercise	Reps	Sets

Additional lifetime/recreational activities? Y N

Type: _____

> *Stay strong, energetic, mentally sharp, and confident, and your age will not define you — or debilitate you.*
> — BOB GREENE

DIET CHECKLIST

Type of Food	Ideal Number of Servings	Breakfast	Lunch	Dinner	Snack(s)	Total Daily Servings
Fruits						
Vegetables (and herbs and spices)						
Grains/legumes/ starchy vegetables						
Milk/yogurt (fat-free or 1%)/soy milk						
High-protein foods						
Nuts/nut butters/seeds						
Healthy fats						
Water						
Superfoods						
Treats/beverages						

Superfoods consumed today (see the list in *20 Years Younger*) _____

_____

Did you take a multivitamin/mineral or other supplement(s)? Y N

SKIN CARE

A.M. Regimen/Products _____

_____

P.M. Regimen/Products _____

_____

Did you apply sunscreen? Y N

SLEEP

GOAL: Hours per night _____

Did you meet this goal today? Y N

WEEKLY SUMMARY

WEEK FOUR   DATE:

PHYSICAL ACTIVITY

Cardiovascular Exercise

GOAL: Minutes (or steps) per week _____

Did you meet or exceed this goal? **Y N**

Strength Training

GOAL: Number of exercises _____ Sets _____
Repetitions per set _____ Days per week _____

Did you meet or exceed this goal? **Y N**

Stretches

GOAL: Stretches _____ Days per week _____

Did you meet or exceed this goal? **Y N**

Core Exercises

GOAL: Exercises _____ Sets _____
Repetitions per set _____ Days per week _____

Did you meet or exceed this goal? **Y N**

Lifetime/Recreational Activities

GOAL: Time(s) per week _____

Did you meet or exceed this goal? **Y N**

DIET

GOAL: Eat the ideal number of servings from each food group —
or get very close — at least five days a week

Did you meet or exceed this goal? **Y N**

GOAL: Eat at least one superfood from each food group daily

Did you meet or exceed this goal? **Y N**

GOAL: Take a multivitamin/mineral or other supplement(s) daily

Did you meet this goal? Y N

SKIN CARE

GOAL: Perform skin care regimen daily in the a.m. and p.m.

Did you meet this goal? Y N

GOAL: Apply sunscreen when needed

Did you meet this goal? Y N

SLEEP

GOAL: Hours per night _____

Did you meet this goal? Y N

Notes

_____
_____
_____
_____
_____
_____
_____
_____
_____
_____
_____
_____
_____
_____
_____
_____
_____
_____
_____
_____
_____
_____
_____

WEEK FIVE

WEEK FIVE   DATE:

Physical Activity

20 YEARS YOUNGER EXERCISE LEVEL: I   II   III

Cardiovascular Exercise

GOAL: Minutes (or steps) per week _____ Today's minutes (or steps) _____

Strength Training

GOAL: Sets _____ Repetitions per set _____ Days per week _____

Strength-Training Exercise	Weight/Resistance	Reps	Sets
_____			
_____			
_____			
_____			
_____			

Stretches

GOAL: Stretches _____ Days per week _____

Stretch

_____   _____

_____   _____

_____

Core Exercises

GOAL: Sets _____ Repetitions per set _____ Days per week _____

Core Exercise	Reps	Sets
_____		
_____		
_____		
_____		
_____		

Additional lifetime/recreational activities? **Y N**

Type: _____

> *If you want your life to come together, you have to start treating yourself better.*
>
> — SARA BAN BREATHNACH

DIET CHECKLIST

Type of Food	Ideal Number of Servings	Breakfast	Lunch	Dinner	Snack(s)	Total Daily Servings
Fruits						
Vegetables (and herbs and spices)						
Grains/legumes/ starchy vegetables						
Milk/yogurt (fat-free or 1%)/soy milk						
High-protein foods						
Nuts/nut butters/seeds						
Healthy fats						
Water						
Superfoods						
Treats/beverages						

Superfoods consumed today (see the list in *20 Years Younger*) _____

_____

Did you take a multivitamin/mineral or other supplement(s)? Y N

SKIN CARE

A.M. Regimen/Products _____

_____

P.M. Regimen/Products _____

_____

Did you apply sunscreen? Y N

SLEEP

GOAL: Hours per night _____

Did you meet this goal today? Y N

WEEK FIVE   DATE:

PHYSICAL ACTIVITY

Cardiovascular Exercise

GOAL: Minutes (or steps) per week _____ Today's minutes (or steps) _____

Strength Training

GOAL: Sets _____ Repetitions per set _____ Days per week _____

Strength-Training Exercise	Weight/Resistance	Reps	Sets

Stretches

GOAL: Stretches _____ Days per week _____

Stretch	

Core Exercises

GOAL: Sets _____ Repetitions per set _____ Days per week _____

Core Exercise	Reps	Sets

Additional lifetime/recreational activities? Y N

Type: _____

> *It is never too late to be what you might have been.*
> — GEORGE ELIOT

DIET CHECKLIST

Type of Food	Ideal Number of Servings	Breakfast	Lunch	Dinner	Snack(s)	Total Daily Servings
Fruits						
Vegetables (and herbs and spices)						
Grains/legumes/ starchy vegetables						
Milk/yogurt (fat-free or 1%)/soy milk						
High-protein foods						
Nuts/nut butters/seeds						
Healthy fats						
Water						
Superfoods						
Treats/beverages						

Superfoods consumed today (see the list in *20 Years Younger*) _____
_____

Did you take a multivitamin/mineral or other supplement(s)? Y N

SKIN CARE

A.M. Regimen/Products _____

_____

P.M. Regimen/Products _____

_____

Did you apply sunscreen? Y N

SLEEP

GOAL: Hours per night _____

Did you meet this goal today? Y N

WEEK FIVE   DATE:

Physical Activity

20 YEARS YOUNGER EXERCISE LEVEL: I   II   III

Cardiovascular Exercise

GOAL: Minutes (or steps) per week _____ Today's minutes (or steps) _____

Strength Training

GOAL: Sets _____ Repetitions per set _____ Days per week _____

Strength-Training Exercise	Weight/Resistance	Reps	Sets

Stretches

GOAL: Stretches _____ Days per week _____

Stretch

_____   _____

_____   _____

_____

Core Exercises

GOAL: Sets _____ Repetitions per set _____ Days per week _____

Core Exercise	Reps	Sets

Additional lifetime/recreational activities? Y N

Type: _____

> *Choice is the engine of our evolution.*
> — GARY ZUKAV

DIET CHECKLIST

Type of Food	Ideal Number of Servings	Breakfast	Lunch	Dinner	Snack(s)	Total Daily Servings
Fruits						
Vegetables (and herbs and spices)						
Grains/legumes/ starchy vegetables						
Milk/yogurt (fat-free or 1%)/soy milk						
High-protein foods						
Nuts/nut butters/seeds						
Healthy fats						
Water						
Superfoods						
Treats/beverages						

Superfoods consumed today (see the list in *20 Years Younger*) _____

_____

Did you take a multivitamin/mineral or other supplement(s)? Y N

SKIN CARE

A.M. Regimen/Products _____

_____

P.M. Regimen/Products _____

_____

Did you apply sunscreen? Y N

SLEEP

GOAL: Hours per night _____

Did you meet this goal today? Y N

WEEK FIVE   DATE: _____

PHYSICAL ACTIVITY

20 YEARS YOUNGER EXERCISE LEVEL: I   II   III

Cardiovascular Exercise

GOAL: Minutes (or steps) per week _____ Today's minutes (or steps) _____

Strength Training

GOAL: Sets _____ Repetitions per set _____ Days per week _____

Strength-Training Exercise	Weight/Resistance	Reps	Sets
_____			
_____			
_____			
_____			
_____			

Stretches

GOAL: Stretches _____ Days per week _____

Stretch	
_____	_____
_____	_____
_____	

Core Exercises

GOAL: Sets _____ Repetitions per set _____ Days per week _____

Core Exercise	Reps	Sets
_____		
_____		
_____		
_____		
_____		

Additional lifetime/recreational activities? **Y N**

Type: _____

> *All excellent things are as difficult as they are rare.*
> — BARUCH BENEDICT DE SPINOZA

DIET CHECKLIST

Type of Food	Ideal Number of Servings	Breakfast	Lunch	Dinner	Snack(s)	Total Daily Servings
Fruits						
Vegetables (and herbs and spices)						
Grains/legumes/ starchy vegetables						
Milk/yogurt (fat-free or 1%)/soy milk						
High-protein foods						
Nuts/nut butters/seeds						
Healthy fats						
Water						
Superfoods						
Treats/beverages						

Superfoods consumed today (see the list in *20 Years Younger*) _____

_____

Did you take a multivitamin/mineral or other supplement(s)? Y N

SKIN CARE

A.M. Regimen/Products _____

_____

P.M. Regimen/Products _____

_____

Did you apply sunscreen? Y N

SLEEP

GOAL: Hours per night _____

Did you meet this goal today? Y N

WEEK FIVE   DATE:

PHYSICAL ACTIVITY

20 YEARS YOUNGER EXERCISE LEVEL: I   II   III

Cardiovascular Exercise

GOAL: Minutes (or steps) per week _____ Today's minutes (or steps) _____

Strength Training

GOAL: Sets _____ Repetitions per set _____ Days per week _____

Strength-Training Exercise	Weight/Resistance	Reps	Sets

Stretches

GOAL: Stretches _____ Days per week _____

Stretch

_____   _____

_____   _____

_____

Core Exercises

GOAL: Sets _____ Repetitions per set _____ Days per week _____

Core Exercise	Reps	Sets

Additional lifetime/recreational activities? Y N

Type: _____

> *We are the hero of our own story.*
> — MARY MCCARTHY

DIET CHECKLIST

Type of Food	Ideal Number of Servings	Breakfast	Lunch	Dinner	Snack(s)	Total Daily Servings
Fruits						
Vegetables (and herbs and spices)						
Grains/legumes/ starchy vegetables						
Milk/yogurt (fat-free or 1%)/soy milk						
High-protein foods						
Nuts/nut butters/seeds						
Healthy fats						
Water						
Superfoods						
Treats/beverages						

Superfoods consumed today (see the list in *20 Years Younger*) _____
_____

Did you take a multivitamin/mineral or other supplement(s)? Y N

SKIN CARE

A.M. Regimen/Products _____
_____

P.M. Regimen/Products _____
_____

Did you apply sunscreen? Y N

SLEEP

GOAL: Hours per night _____

Did you meet this goal today? Y N

WEEK FIVE   DATE:

Physical Activity

20 YEARS YOUNGER EXERCISE LEVEL: I   II   III

Cardiovascular Exercise

GOAL: Minutes (or steps) per week _____ Today's minutes (or steps) _____

Strength Training

GOAL: Sets _____ Repetitions per set _____ Days per week _____

Strength-Training Exercise	Weight/Resistance	Reps	Sets

Stretches

GOAL: Stretches _____ Days per week _____

Stretch

_____   _____

_____   _____

_____

Core Exercises

GOAL: Sets _____ Repetitions per set _____ Days per week _____

Core Exercise	Reps	Sets

Additional lifetime/recreational activities? Y N

Type: _____

> *Nothing will ever be attempted if all possible objections must first be overcome.*
> — SAMUEL JOHNSON

DIET CHECKLIST

Type of Food	Ideal Number of Servings	Breakfast	Lunch	Dinner	Snack(s)	Total Daily Servings
Fruits						
Vegetables (and herbs and spices)						
Grains/legumes/ starchy vegetables						
Milk/yogurt (fat-free or 1%)/soy milk						
High-protein foods						
Nuts/nut butters/seeds						
Healthy fats						
Water						
Superfoods						
Treats/beverages						

Superfoods consumed today (see the list in *20 Years Younger*) _____

_____

Did you take a multivitamin/mineral or other supplement(s)? Y N

SKIN CARE

A.M. Regimen/Products _____

_____

P.M. Regimen/Products _____

_____

Did you apply sunscreen? Y N

SLEEP

GOAL: Hours per night _____

Did you meet this goal today? Y N

WEEK FIVE   DATE:

Physical Activity

20 YEARS YOUNGER EXERCISE LEVEL: I   II   III

Cardiovascular Exercise

GOAL: Minutes (or steps) per week _____ Today's minutes (or steps) _____

Strength Training

GOAL: Sets _____ Repetitions per set _____ Days per week _____

Strength-Training Exercise	Weight/Resistance	Reps	Sets
_____			
_____			
_____			
_____			
_____			
_____			

Stretches

GOAL: Stretches _____ Days per week _____

Stretch	
_____	_____
_____	_____
_____	

Core Exercises

GOAL: Sets _____ Repetitions per set _____ Days per week _____

Core Exercise	Reps	Sets
_____		
_____		
_____		
_____		
_____		
_____		

Additional lifetime/recreational activities? Y N

Type: _____

> *The body is shaped, disciplined, honored, and in time, trusted.*
> — MARTHA GRAHAM

DIET CHECKLIST

Type of Food	Ideal Number of Servings	Breakfast	Lunch	Dinner	Snack(s)	Total Daily Servings
Fruits						
Vegetables (and herbs and spices)						
Grains/legumes/ starchy vegetables						
Milk/yogurt (fat-free or 1%)/soy milk						
High-protein foods						
Nuts/nut butters/seeds						
Healthy fats						
Water						
Superfoods						
Treats/beverages						

Superfoods consumed today (see the list in *20 Years Younger*) _____

_____

Did you take a multivitamin/mineral or other supplement(s)? Y N

SKIN CARE

A.M. Regimen/Products _____

_____

P.M. Regimen/Products _____

_____

Did you apply sunscreen? Y N

SLEEP

GOAL: Hours per night _____

Did you meet this goal today? Y N

WEEKLY SUMMARY

WEEK FIVE
DATE:

20 YEARS YOUNGER EXERCISE LEVEL: I   II   III

PHYSICAL ACTIVITY

Cardiovascular Exercise

GOAL: Minutes (or steps) per week _____

Did you meet or exceed this goal? Y N

Strength Training

GOAL: Number of exercises _____ Sets _____
        Repetitions per set _____ Days per week _____

Did you meet or exceed this goal? Y N

Stretches

GOAL: Stretches _____ Days per week _____

Did you meet or exceed this goal? Y N

Core Exercises

GOAL: Exercises _____ Sets _____
        Repetitions per set _____ Days per week _____

Did you meet or exceed this goal? Y N

Lifetime/Recreational Activities

GOAL: Time(s) per week _____

Did you meet or exceed this goal? Y N

DIET

GOAL: Eat the ideal number of servings from each food group—
        or get very close—at least five days a week

Did you meet or exceed this goal? Y N

GOAL: Eat at least one superfood from each food group daily

Did you meet or exceed this goal? Y N

GOAL: Take a multivitamin/mineral or other supplement(s) daily

Did you meet this goal? Y N

Skin Care

GOAL: Perform skin care regimen daily in the a.m. and p.m.

Did you meet this goal? Y N

GOAL: Apply sunscreen when needed

Did you meet this goal? Y N

Sleep

GOAL: Hours per night _____

Did you meet this goal? Y N

Notes

_____

_____

_____

_____

_____

_____

_____

_____

_____

_____

_____

_____

_____

_____

_____

_____

_____

_____

_____

_____

_____

_____

_____

_____

_____

WEEK SIX

WEEK SIX DATE:

PHYSICAL ACTIVITY

20 YEARS YOUNGER EXERCISE LEVEL: I   II   III

Cardiovascular Exercise

GOAL: Minutes (or steps) per week _____ Today's minutes (or steps) _____

Strength Training

GOAL: Sets _____ Repetitions per set _____ Days per week _____

Strength-Training Exercise	Weight/Resistance	Reps	Sets

Stretches

GOAL: Stretches _____ Days per week _____

Stretch

_____   _____

_____   _____

_____

Core Exercises

GOAL: Sets _____ Repetitions per set _____ Days per week _____

Core Exercise	Reps	Sets

Additional lifetime/recreational activities? Y N

Type: _____

DIET CHECKLIST

Type of Food	Ideal Number of Servings	Breakfast	Lunch	Dinner	Snack(s)	Total Daily Servings
Fruits						
Vegetables (and herbs and spices)						
Grains/legumes/ starchy vegetables						
Milk/yogurt (fat-free or 1%)/soy milk						
High-protein foods						
Nuts/nut butters/seeds						
Healthy fats						
Water						
Superfoods						
Treats/beverages						

Superfoods consumed today (see the list in *20 Years Younger*) _____

_____

Did you take a multivitamin/mineral or other supplement(s)? Y N

SKIN CARE

A.M. Regimen/Products _____

_____

P.M. Regimen/Products _____

_____

Did you apply sunscreen? Y N

SLEEP

GOAL: Hours per night _____

Did you meet this goal today? Y N

WEEK SIX   DATE:

Physical Activity

20 YEARS YOUNGER EXERCISE LEVEL: I   II   III

Cardiovascular Exercise

GOAL: Minutes (or steps) per week _____ Today's minutes (or steps) _____

Strength Training

GOAL: Sets _____ Repetitions per set _____ Days per week _____

Strength-Training Exercise	Weight/Resistance	Reps	Sets

Stretches

GOAL: Stretches _____ Days per week _____

Stretch

Core Exercises

GOAL: Sets _____ Repetitions per set _____ Days per week _____

Core Exercise	Reps	Sets

Additional lifetime/recreational activities? Y N

Type: _____

DIET CHECKLIST

Type of Food	Ideal Number of Servings	Breakfast	Lunch	Dinner	Snack(s)	Total Daily Servings
Fruits						
Vegetables (and herbs and spices)						
Grains/legumes/ starchy vegetables						
Milk/yogurt (fat-free or 1%)/soy milk						
High-protein foods						
Nuts/nut butters/seeds						
Healthy fats						
Water						
Superfoods						
Treats/beverages						

Superfoods consumed today (see the list in *20 Years Younger*) _____

_____

Did you take a multivitamin/mineral or other supplement(s)? Y N

SKIN CARE

A.M. Regimen/Products _____

_____

P.M. Regimen/Products _____

_____

Did you apply sunscreen? Y N

SLEEP

GOAL: Hours per night _____

Did you meet this goal today? Y N

WEEK SIX DATE:

Physical Activity

20 YEARS YOUNGER EXERCISE LEVEL: I   II   III

Cardiovascular Exercise

GOAL: Minutes (or steps) per week _____ Today's minutes (or steps) _____

Strength Training

GOAL: Sets _____ Repetitions per set _____ Days per week _____

Strength-Training Exercise	Weight/Resistance	Reps	Sets

Stretches

GOAL: Stretches _____ Days per week _____

Stretch

_____   _____

_____   _____

_____

Core Exercises

GOAL: Sets _____ Repetitions per set _____ Days per week _____

Core Exercise	Reps	Sets

Additional lifetime/recreational activities? Y N

Type: _____

> *Things do not change; we change.*
> — Henry David Thoreau

Diet Checklist

Type of Food	Ideal Number of Servings	Breakfast	Lunch	Dinner	Snack(s)	Total Daily Servings
Fruits						
Vegetables (and herbs and spices)						
Grains/legumes/ starchy vegetables						
Milk/yogurt (fat-free or 1%)/soy milk						
High-protein foods						
Nuts/nut butters/seeds						
Healthy fats						
Water						
Superfoods						
Treats/beverages						

Superfoods consumed today (see the list in *20 Years Younger*) _____
_____

Did you take a multivitamin/mineral or other supplement(s)? Y N

Skin Care

A.M. Regimen/Products _____
_____

P.M. Regimen/Products _____
_____

Did you apply sunscreen? Y N

Sleep

GOAL: Hours per night _____

Did you meet this goal today? Y N

WEEK SIX   DATE: _____

PHYSICAL ACTIVITY

20 YEARS YOUNGER EXERCISE LEVEL: I   II   III

Cardiovascular Exercise

GOAL: Minutes (or steps) per week _____ Today's minutes (or steps) _____

Strength Training

GOAL: Sets _____ Repetitions per set _____ Days per week _____

Strength-Training Exercise	Weight/Resistance	Reps	Sets

Stretches

GOAL: Stretches _____ Days per week _____

Stretch

_____   _____

_____   _____

_____

Core Exercises

GOAL: Sets _____ Repetitions per set _____ Days per week _____

Core Exercise	Reps	Sets

Additional lifetime/recreational activities? **Y   N**

Type: _____

> *Any little experimenting in self-nurturance is*
> *very frightening for most of us.*
> — JULIA CAMERON

DIET CHECKLIST

Type of Food	Ideal Number of Servings	Breakfast	Lunch	Dinner	Snack(s)	Total Daily Servings
Fruits						
Vegetables (and herbs and spices)						
Grains/legumes/ starchy vegetables						
Milk/yogurt (fat-free or 1%)/soy milk						
High-protein foods						
Nuts/nut butters/seeds						
Healthy fats						
Water						
Superfoods						
Treats/beverages						

Superfoods consumed today (see the list in *20 Years Younger*) _____

_____

Did you take a multivitamin/mineral or other supplement(s)? **Y N**

SKIN CARE

A.M. Regimen/Products _____

_____

P.M. Regimen/Products _____

_____

Did you apply sunscreen? **Y N**

SLEEP

GOAL: Hours per night _____

Did you meet this goal today? **Y N**

WEEK SIX   DATE:

Physical Activity

20 YEARS YOUNGER EXERCISE LEVEL: I   II   III

Cardiovascular Exercise

GOAL: Minutes (or steps) per week _____ Today's minutes (or steps) _____

Strength Training

GOAL: Sets _____ Repetitions per set _____ Days per week _____

Strength-Training Exercise	Weight/Resistance	Reps	Sets

Stretches

GOAL: Stretches _____ Days per week _____

Stretch

_____   _____

_____   _____

_____

Core Exercises

GOAL: Sets _____ Repetitions per set _____ Days per week _____

Core Exercise	Reps	Sets

Additional lifetime/recreational activities? **Y N**

Type: _____

> *A man should always consider how much he has more than he wants; and secondly, how much more unhappy he might be than he really is.*
>
> — JOSEPH ADDISON

DIET CHECKLIST

Type of Food	Ideal Number of Servings	Breakfast	Lunch	Dinner	Snack(s)	Total Daily Servings
Fruits						
Vegetables (and herbs and spices)						
Grains/legumes/ starchy vegetables						
Milk/yogurt (fat-free or 1%)/soy milk						
High-protein foods						
Nuts/nut butters/seeds						
Healthy fats						
Water						
Superfoods						
Treats/beverages						

Superfoods consumed today (see the list in *20 Years Younger*) _____

_____

Did you take a multivitamin/mineral or other supplement(s)? Y N

SKIN CARE

A.M. Regimen/Products _____

_____

P.M. Regimen/Products _____

_____

Did you apply sunscreen? Y N

SLEEP

GOAL: Hours per night _____

Did you meet this goal today? Y N

WEEK SIX   DATE:

Physical Activity

20 YEARS YOUNGER EXERCISE LEVEL: I   II   III

Cardiovascular Exercise

GOAL: Minutes (or steps) per week _____ Today's minutes (or steps) _____

Strength Training

GOAL: Sets _____ Repetitions per set _____ Days per week _____

Strength-Training Exercise	Weight/Resistance	Reps	Sets
_____			
_____			
_____			
_____			
_____			
_____			

Stretches

GOAL: Stretches _____ Days per week _____

Stretch

_____   _____

_____   _____

_____

Core Exercises

GOAL: Sets _____ Repetitions per set _____ Days per week _____

Core Exercise	Reps	Sets
_____		
_____		
_____		
_____		
_____		
_____		

Additional lifetime/recreational activities? **Y N**

Type: _____

> *If we could give every individual the right amount of*
> *nourishment and exercise, not too little and not too much,*
> *we would have found the safest way to health.*
>
> — Hippocrates

DIET CHECKLIST

Type of Food	Ideal Number of Servings	Breakfast	Lunch	Dinner	Snack(s)	Total Daily Servings
Fruits						
Vegetables (and herbs and spices)						
Grains/legumes/ starchy vegetables						
Milk/yogurt (fat-free or 1%)/soy milk						
High-protein foods						
Nuts/nut butters/seeds						
Healthy fats						
Water						
Superfoods						
Treats/beverages						

Superfoods consumed today (see the list in *20 Years Younger*) _____

_____

Did you take a multivitamin/mineral or other supplement(s)? Y N

SKIN CARE

A.M. Regimen/Products _____

_____

P.M. Regimen/Products _____

_____

Did you apply sunscreen? Y N

SLEEP

GOAL: Hours per night _____

Did you meet this goal today? Y N

WEEK SIX   DATE:

Physical Activity

20 YEARS YOUNGER EXERCISE LEVEL: I   II   III

Cardiovascular Exercise

GOAL: Minutes (or steps) per week _____ Today's minutes (or steps) _____

Strength Training

GOAL: Sets _____ Repetitions per set _____ Days per week _____

Strength-Training Exercise	Weight/Resistance	Reps	Sets

Stretches

GOAL: Stretches _____ Days per week _____

Stretch

_____   _____
_____   _____
_____

Core Exercises

GOAL: Sets _____ Repetitions per set _____ Days per week _____

Core Exercise	Reps	Sets

Additional lifetime/recreational activities? Y N

Type: _____

DIET CHECKLIST

Type of Food	Ideal Number of Servings	Breakfast	Lunch	Dinner	Snack(s)	Total Daily Servings
Fruits						
Vegetables (and herbs and spices)						
Grains/legumes/ starchy vegetables						
Milk/yogurt (fat-free or 1%)/soy milk						
High-protein foods						
Nuts/nut butters/seeds						
Healthy fats						
Water						
Superfoods						
Treats/beverages						

Superfoods consumed today (see the list in *20 Years Younger*) _____

_____

Did you take a multivitamin/mineral or other supplement(s)? Y N

SKIN CARE

A.M. Regimen/Products _____

_____

P.M. Regimen/Products _____

_____

Did you apply sunscreen? Y N

SLEEP

GOAL: Hours per night _____

Did you meet this goal today? Y N

WEEKLY SUMMARY

WEEK SIX   DATE:

20 YEARS YOUNGER EXERCISE LEVEL: I   II   III

Physical Activity

Cardiovascular Exercise

GOAL: Minutes (or steps) per week _____

Did you meet or exceed this goal? Y N

Strength Training

GOAL: Number of exercises _____ Sets _____

Repetitions per set _____ Days per week _____

Did you meet or exceed this goal? Y N

Stretches

GOAL: Stretches _____ Days per week _____

Did you meet or exceed this goal? Y N

Core Exercises

GOAL: Exercises _____ Sets _____

Repetitions per set _____ Days per week _____

Did you meet or exceed this goal? Y N

Lifetime/Recreational Activities

GOAL: Time(s) per week _____

Did you meet or exceed this goal? Y N

Diet

GOAL: Eat the ideal number of servings from each food group —
or get very close — at least five days a week

Did you meet or exceed this goal? Y N

GOAL: Eat at least one superfood from each food group daily

Did you meet or exceed this goal? Y N

GOAL: Take a multivitamin/mineral or other supplement(s) daily

Did you meet this goal? Y N

Skin Care

GOAL: Perform skin care regimen daily in the a.m. and p.m.

Did you meet this goal? Y N

GOAL: Apply sunscreen when needed

Did you meet this goal? Y N

Sleep

GOAL: Hours per night _____

Did you meet this goal? Y N

Notes

_____
_____
_____
_____
_____
_____
_____
_____
_____
_____
_____
_____
_____
_____
_____
_____
_____
_____
_____
_____
_____
_____
_____

WEEK SEVEN

WEEK SEVEN   DATE: _____

Physical Activity

20 YEARS YOUNGER EXERCISE LEVEL: I   II   III

Cardiovascular Exercise

GOAL: Minutes (or steps) per week _____ Today's minutes (or steps) _____

Strength Training

GOAL: Sets _____ Repetitions per set _____ Days per week _____

Strength-Training Exercise	Weight/Resistance	Reps	Sets
_____			
_____			
_____			
_____			
_____			

Stretches

GOAL: Stretches _____ Days per week _____

Stretch	
_____	_____
_____	_____
_____	

Core Exercises

GOAL: Sets _____ Repetitions per set _____ Days per week _____

Core Exercise	Reps	Sets
_____		
_____		
_____		
_____		
_____		

Additional lifetime/recreational activities? **Y N**

Type: _____

> *We were meant to move.*
> — BOB GREENE

DIET CHECKLIST

Type of Food	Ideal Number of Servings	Breakfast	Lunch	Dinner	Snack(s)	Total Daily Servings
Fruits						
Vegetables (and herbs and spices)						
Grains/legumes/ starchy vegetables						
Milk/yogurt (fat-free or 1%)/soy milk						
High-protein foods						
Nuts/nut butters/seeds						
Healthy fats						
Water						
Superfoods						
Treats/beverages						

Superfoods consumed today (see the list in *20 Years Younger*) _____
_____

Did you take a multivitamin/mineral or other supplement(s)? Y N

SKIN CARE

A.M. Regimen/Products _____
_____

P.M. Regimen/Products _____
_____

Did you apply sunscreen? Y N

SLEEP

GOAL: Hours per night _____

Did you meet this goal today? Y N

WEEK SEVEN   DATE: _____

PHYSICAL ACTIVITY

20 YEARS YOUNGER EXERCISE LEVEL: I   II   III

Cardiovascular Exercise

GOAL: Minutes (or steps) per week _____ Today's minutes (or steps) _____

Strength Training

GOAL: Sets _____ Repetitions per set _____ Days per week _____

Strength-Training Exercise	Weight/Resistance	Reps	Sets

Stretches

GOAL: Stretches _____ Days per week _____

Stretch	

Core Exercises

GOAL: Sets _____ Repetitions per set _____ Days per week _____

Core Exercise	Reps	Sets

Additional lifetime/recreational activities? Y N

Type: _____

> *Your real influence is measured by your treatment of yourself.*
>
> — A. BRONSON ALCOTT

DIET CHECKLIST

Type of Food	Ideal Number of Servings	Breakfast	Lunch	Dinner	Snack(s)	Total Daily Servings
Fruits						
Vegetables (and herbs and spices)						
Grains/legumes/ starchy vegetables						
Milk/yogurt (fat-free or 1%)/soy milk						
High-protein foods						
Nuts/nut butters/seeds						
Healthy fats						
Water						
Superfoods						
Treats/beverages						

Superfoods consumed today (see the list in *20 Years Younger*) _____

_____

Did you take a multivitamin/mineral or other supplement(s)? Y N

SKIN CARE

A.M. Regimen/Products _____

_____

P.M. Regimen/Products _____

_____

Did you apply sunscreen? Y N

SLEEP

GOAL: Hours per night _____

Did you meet this goal today? Y N

WEEK SEVEN   DATE: _____

Physical Activity

20 YEARS YOUNGER EXERCISE LEVEL: I   II   III

Cardiovascular Exercise

GOAL: Minutes (or steps) per week _____ Today's minutes (or steps) _____

Strength Training

GOAL: Sets _____ Repetitions per set _____ Days per week _____

Strength-Training Exercise	Weight/Resistance	Reps	Sets

Stretches

GOAL: Stretches _____ Days per week _____

Stretch

_____   _____

_____   _____

_____

Core Exercises

GOAL: Sets _____ Repetitions per set _____ Days per week _____

Core Exercise	Reps	Sets

Additional lifetime/recreational activities? Y N

Type: _____

> *Live now, believe me, wait not till tomorrow;*
> *gather the roses of life today.*
> — PIERRE DE RONSARD

DIET CHECKLIST

Type of Food	Ideal Number of Servings	Breakfast	Lunch	Dinner	Snack(s)	Total Daily Servings
Fruits						
Vegetables (and herbs and spices)						
Grains/legumes/ starchy vegetables						
Milk/yogurt (fat-free or 1%)/soy milk						
High-protein foods						
Nuts/nut butters/seeds						
Healthy fats						
Water						
Superfoods						
Treats/beverages						

Superfoods consumed today (see the list in *20 Years Younger*) _____
_____

Did you take a multivitamin/mineral or other supplement(s)? Y N

SKIN CARE

A.M. Regimen/Products _____
_____

P.M. Regimen/Products _____
_____

Did you apply sunscreen? Y N

SLEEP

GOAL: Hours per night _____

Did you meet this goal today? Y N

WEEK SEVEN   DATE:

Physical Activity

20 YEARS YOUNGER EXERCISE LEVEL: I   II   III

Cardiovascular Exercise

GOAL: Minutes (or steps) per week _____ Today's minutes (or steps) _____

Strength Training

GOAL: Sets _____ Repetitions per set _____ Days per week _____

Strength-Training Exercise	Weight/Resistance	Reps	Sets

Stretches

GOAL: Stretches _____ Days per week _____

Stretch

_____   _____

_____   _____

_____

Core Exercises

GOAL: Sets _____ Repetitions per set _____ Days per week _____

Core Exercise	Reps	Sets

Additional lifetime/recreational activities? Y N

Type: _____

> *Give yourself the gift of a good night's sleep.*
> — Ronald Kotler, MD

Diet Checklist

Type of Food	Ideal Number of Servings	Breakfast	Lunch	Dinner	Snack(s)	Total Daily Servings
Fruits						
Vegetables (and herbs and spices)						
Grains/legumes/ starchy vegetables						
Milk/yogurt (fat-free or 1%)/soy milk						
High-protein foods						
Nuts/nut butters/seeds						
Healthy fats						
Water						
Superfoods						
Treats/beverages						

Superfoods consumed today (see the list in *20 Years Younger*) _____

Did you take a multivitamin/mineral or other supplement(s)? Y N

Skin Care

A.M. Regimen/Products _____

_____

P.M. Regimen/Products _____

_____

Did you apply sunscreen? Y N

Sleep

GOAL: Hours per night _____

Did you meet this goal today? Y N

WEEK SEVEN   DATE: _____

Physical Activity

20 YEARS YOUNGER EXERCISE LEVEL: I   II   III

Cardiovascular Exercise

GOAL: Minutes (or steps) per week _____ Today's minutes (or steps) _____

Strength Training

GOAL: Sets _____ Repetitions per set _____ Days per week _____

Strength-Training Exercise	Weight/Resistance	Reps	Sets

Stretches

GOAL: Stretches _____ Days per week _____

Stretch

Core Exercises

GOAL: Sets _____ Repetitions per set _____ Days per week _____

Core Exercise	Reps	Sets

Additional lifetime/recreational activities? **Y N**

Type: _____

Diet Checklist

Type of Food	Ideal Number of Servings	Breakfast	Lunch	Dinner	Snack(s)	Total Daily Servings
Fruits						
Vegetables (and herbs and spices)						
Grains/legumes/ starchy vegetables						
Milk/yogurt (fat-free or 1%)/soy milk						
High-protein foods						
Nuts/nut butters/seeds						
Healthy fats						
Water						
Superfoods						
Treats/beverages						

Superfoods consumed today (see the list in *20 Years Younger*) _____

_____

Did you take a multivitamin/mineral or other supplement(s)? Y N

Skin Care

A.M. Regimen/Products _____

_____

P.M. Regimen/Products _____

_____

Did you apply sunscreen? Y N

Sleep

GOAL: Hours per night _____

Did you meet this goal today? Y N

WEEK SEVEN   DATE: _____

Physical Activity

20 YEARS YOUNGER EXERCISE LEVEL: I   II   III

Cardiovascular Exercise

GOAL: Minutes (or steps) per week _____ Today's minutes (or steps) _____

Strength Training

GOAL: Sets _____ Repetitions per set _____ Days per week _____

Strength-Training Exercise	Weight/Resistance	Reps	Sets
_____			
_____			
_____			
_____			
_____			
_____			

Stretches

GOAL: Stretches _____ Days per week _____

Stretch

_____   _____

_____   _____

_____

Core Exercises

GOAL: Sets _____ Repetitions per set _____ Days per week _____

Core Exercise	Reps	Sets
_____		
_____		
_____		
_____		
_____		
_____		

Additional lifetime/recreational activities? **Y N**

Type: _____

> *The reward of a thing well done is to have done it.*
> — RALPH WALDO EMERSON, *ESSAYS*

DIET CHECKLIST

Type of Food	Ideal Number of Servings	Breakfast	Lunch	Dinner	Snack(s)	Total Daily Servings
Fruits						
Vegetables (and herbs and spices)						
Grains/legumes/ starchy vegetables						
Milk/yogurt (fat-free or 1%)/soy milk						
High-protein foods						
Nuts/nut butters/seeds						
Healthy fats						
Water						
Superfoods						
Treats/beverages						

Superfoods consumed today (see the list in *20 Years Younger*) _____

_____

Did you take a multivitamin/mineral or other supplement(s)? Y N

SKIN CARE

A.M. Regimen/Products _____

_____

P.M. Regimen/Products _____

_____

Did you apply sunscreen? Y N

SLEEP

GOAL: Hours per night _____

Did you meet this goal today? Y N

WEEK SEVEN   DATE:

Physical Activity

20 YEARS YOUNGER EXERCISE LEVEL: I   II   III

Cardiovascular Exercise

GOAL: Minutes (or steps) per week _____ Today's minutes (or steps) _____

Strength Training

GOAL: Sets _____ Repetitions per set _____ Days per week _____

Strength-Training Exercise	Weight/Resistance	Reps	Sets

Stretches

GOAL: Stretches _____ Days per week _____

Stretch

_____   _____

_____   _____

_____

Core Exercises

GOAL: Sets _____ Repetitions per set _____ Days per week _____

Core Exercise	Reps	Sets

Additional lifetime/recreational activities? Y N

Type: _____

> *May you live all the days of your life.*
> — JONATHAN SWIFT, *POLITE CONVERSATION*

DIET CHECKLIST

Type of Food	Ideal Number of Servings	Breakfast	Lunch	Dinner	Snack(s)	Total Daily Servings
Fruits						
Vegetables (and herbs and spices)						
Grains/legumes/ starchy vegetables						
Milk/yogurt (fat-free or 1%)/soy milk						
High-protein foods						
Nuts/nut butters/seeds						
Healthy fats						
Water						
Superfoods						
Treats/beverages						

Superfoods consumed today (see the list in *20 Years Younger*) _____

_____

Did you take a multivitamin/mineral or other supplement(s)? Y N

SKIN CARE

A.M. Regimen/Products _____

_____

P.M. Regimen/Products _____

_____

Did you apply sunscreen? Y N

SLEEP

GOAL: Hours per night _____

Did you meet this goal today? Y N

WEEKLY SUMMARY

WEEK SEVEN

DATE: _____

20 YEARS YOUNGER EXERCISE LEVEL: I   II   III

PHYSICAL ACTIVITY

Cardiovascular Exercise

GOAL: Minutes (or steps) per week _____

Did you meet or exceed this goal? Y N

Strength Training

GOAL: Number of exercises _____ Sets _____

Repetitions per set _____ Days per week _____

Did you meet or exceed this goal? Y N

Stretches

GOAL: Stretches _____ Days per week _____

Did you meet or exceed this goal? Y N

Core Exercises

GOAL: Exercises _____ Sets _____

Repetitions per set _____ Days per week _____

Did you meet or exceed this goal? Y N

Lifetime/Recreational Activities

GOAL: Time(s) per week _____

Did you meet or exceed this goal? Y N

DIET

GOAL: Eat the ideal number of servings from each food group —
or get very close — at least five days a week

Did you meet or exceed this goal? Y N

GOAL: Eat at least one superfood from each food group daily

Did you meet or exceed this goal? Y N

GOAL: Take a multivitamin/mineral or other supplement(s) daily

Did you meet this goal? Y N

Skin Care

GOAL: Perform skin care regimen daily in the a.m. and p.m.

Did you meet this goal? Y N

GOAL: Apply sunscreen when needed

Did you meet this goal? Y N

Sleep

GOAL: Hours per night _____

Did you meet this goal? Y N

Notes

_____
_____
_____
_____
_____
_____
_____
_____
_____
_____
_____
_____
_____
_____
_____
_____
_____
_____
_____
_____
_____
_____
_____
_____
_____
_____

WEEK EIGHT

WEEK EIGHT   DATE: _____

PHYSICAL ACTIVITY

20 YEARS YOUNGER EXERCISE LEVEL: I   II   III

Cardiovascular Exercise

GOAL: Minutes (or steps) per week _____ Today's minutes (or steps) _____

Strength Training

GOAL: Sets _____ Repetitions per set _____ Days per week _____

Strength-Training Exercise	Weight/Resistance	Reps	Sets
_____			
_____			
_____			
_____			
_____			
_____			

Stretches

GOAL: Stretches _____ Days per week _____

Stretch	
_____	_____
_____	_____
_____	

Core Exercises

GOAL: Sets _____ Repetitions per set _____ Days per week _____

Core Exercise	Reps	Sets
_____		
_____		
_____		
_____		
_____		
_____		

Additional lifetime/recreational activities? **Y N**

Type: _____

> *If I had to boil down all of the sociopsychological factors that help you age gracefully into one word, that word would be* happiness.
> — BOB GREENE

DIET CHECKLIST

Type of Food	Ideal Number of Servings	Breakfast	Lunch	Dinner	Snack(s)	Total Daily Servings
Fruits						
Vegetables (and herbs and spices)						
Grains/legumes/ starchy vegetables						
Milk/yogurt (fat-free or 1%)/soy milk						
High-protein foods						
Nuts/nut butters/seeds						
Healthy fats						
Water						
Superfoods						
Treats/beverages						

Superfoods consumed today (see the list in *20 Years Younger*) _____
_____

Did you take a multivitamin/mineral or other supplement(s)? Y N

SKIN CARE

A.M. Regimen/Products _____
_____

P.M. Regimen/Products _____
_____

Did you apply sunscreen? Y N

SLEEP

GOAL: Hours per night _____

Did you meet this goal today? Y N

WEEK EIGHT   DATE: _____

PHYSICAL ACTIVITY

20 YEARS YOUNGER EXERCISE LEVEL: I   II   III

Cardiovascular Exercise

GOAL: Minutes (or steps) per week _____ Today's minutes (or steps) _____

Strength Training

GOAL: Sets _____ Repetitions per set _____ Days per week _____

Strength-Training Exercise	Weight/Resistance	Reps	Sets

Stretches

GOAL: Stretches _____ Days per week _____

Stretch

_____   _____

_____   _____

_____

Core Exercises

GOAL: Sets _____ Repetitions per set _____ Days per week _____

Core Exercise	Reps	Sets

Additional lifetime/recreational activities? Y N

Type: _____

> *We know nothing of tomorrow; our business*
> *is to be good and happy today.*
> — SYDNEY SMITH, *LADY HOLLAND'S MEMOIR*

DIET CHECKLIST

Type of Food	Ideal Number of Servings	Breakfast	Lunch	Dinner	Snack(s)	Total Daily Servings
Fruits						
Vegetables (and herbs and spices)						
Grains/legumes/ starchy vegetables						
Milk/yogurt (fat-free or 1%)/soy milk						
High-protein foods						
Nuts/nut butters/seeds						
Healthy fats						
Water						
Superfoods						
Treats/beverages						

Superfoods consumed today (see the list in *20 Years Younger*) _____

_____

Did you take a multivitamin/mineral or other supplement(s)? Y N

SKIN CARE

A.M. Regimen/Products _____

_____

P.M. Regimen/Products _____

_____

Did you apply sunscreen? Y N

SLEEP

GOAL: Hours per night _____

Did you meet this goal today? Y N

WEEK EIGHT   DATE:

Physical Activity

20 YEARS YOUNGER EXERCISE LEVEL: I   II   III

Cardiovascular Exercise

GOAL: Minutes (or steps) per week _____ Today's minutes (or steps) _____

Strength Training

GOAL: Sets _____ Repetitions per set _____ Days per week _____

Strength-Training Exercise	Weight/Resistance	Reps	Sets

Stretches

GOAL: Stretches _____ Days per week _____

Stretch	

Core Exercises

GOAL: Sets _____ Repetitions per set _____ Days per week _____

Core Exercise	Reps	Sets

Additional lifetime/recreational activities? Y N

Type: _____

DIET CHECKLIST

Type of Food	Ideal Number of Servings	Breakfast	Lunch	Dinner	Snack(s)	Total Daily Servings
Fruits						
Vegetables (and herbs and spices)						
Grains/legumes/ starchy vegetables						
Milk/yogurt (fat-free or 1%)/soy milk						
High-protein foods						
Nuts/nut butters/seeds						
Healthy fats						
Water						
Superfoods						
Treats/beverages						

Superfoods consumed today (see the list in *20 Years Younger*) _____

_____

Did you take a multivitamin/mineral or other supplement(s)? Y N

SKIN CARE

A.M. Regimen/Products _____

_____

P.M. Regimen/Products _____

_____

Did you apply sunscreen? Y N

SLEEP

GOAL: Hours per night _____

Did you meet this goal today? Y N

WEEK EIGHT   DATE:

Physical Activity

20 YEARS YOUNGER EXERCISE LEVEL: I   II   III

Cardiovascular Exercise

GOAL: Minutes (or steps) per week _____ Today's minutes (or steps) _____

Strength Training

GOAL: Sets _____ Repetitions per set _____ Days per week _____

Strength-Training Exercise	Weight/Resistance	Reps	Sets
_____			
_____			
_____			
_____			
_____			
_____			

Stretches

GOAL: Stretches _____ Days per week _____

Stretch	
_____	_____
_____	_____
_____	

Core Exercises

GOAL: Sets _____ Repetitions per set _____ Days per week _____

Core Exercise	Reps	Sets
_____		
_____		
_____		
_____		
_____		
_____		

Additional lifetime/recreational activities? **Y N**

Type: _____

> *There is no duty we so much underrate as the duty of being happy.*
>
> — ROBERT LOUIS STEVENSON, *VIRGINIBUS PUERISQUE*

DIET CHECKLIST

Type of Food	Ideal Number of Servings	Breakfast	Lunch	Dinner	Snack(s)	Total Daily Servings
Fruits						
Vegetables (and herbs and spices)						
Grains/legumes/ starchy vegetables						
Milk/yogurt (fat-free or 1%)/soy milk						
High-protein foods						
Nuts/nut butters/seeds						
Healthy fats						
Water						
Superfoods						
Treats/beverages						

Superfoods consumed today (see the list in *20 Years Younger*) _____

_____

Did you take a multivitamin/mineral or other supplement(s)? Y N

SKIN CARE

A.M. Regimen/Products _____

_____

P.M. Regimen/Products _____

_____

Did you apply sunscreen? Y N

SLEEP

GOAL: Hours per night _____

Did you meet this goal today? Y N

WEEK EIGHT   DATE:

PHYSICAL ACTIVITY

20 YEARS YOUNGER EXERCISE LEVEL: I   II   III

Cardiovascular Exercise

GOAL: Minutes (or steps) per week _____ Today's minutes (or steps) _____

Strength Training

GOAL: Sets _____ Repetitions per set _____ Days per week _____

Strength-Training Exercise	Weight/Resistance	Reps	Sets
_____			
_____			
_____			
_____			
_____			

Stretches

GOAL: Stretches _____ Days per week _____

Stretch

_____   _____

_____   _____

_____

Core Exercises

GOAL: Sets _____ Repetitions per set _____ Days per week _____

Core Exercise	Reps	Sets
_____		
_____		
_____		
_____		
_____		

Additional lifetime/recreational activities? **Y   N**

Type: _____

DIET CHECKLIST

Type of Food	Ideal Number of Servings	Breakfast	Lunch	Dinner	Snack(s)	Total Daily Servings
Fruits						
Vegetables (and herbs and spices)						
Grains/legumes/ starchy vegetables						
Milk/yogurt (fat-free or 1%)/soy milk						
High-protein foods						
Nuts/nut butters/seeds						
Healthy fats						
Water						
Superfoods						
Treats/beverages						

Superfoods consumed today (see the list in *20 Years Younger*) _____

_____

Did you take a multivitamin/mineral or other supplement(s)? Y N

SKIN CARE

A.M. Regimen/Products _____

_____

P.M. Regimen/Products _____

_____

Did you apply sunscreen? Y N

SLEEP

GOAL: Hours per night _____

Did you meet this goal today? Y N

WEEK EIGHT

DATE: _____

Physical Activity

20 YEARS YOUNGER EXERCISE LEVEL: I   II   III

Cardiovascular Exercise

GOAL: Minutes (or steps) per week _____ Today's minutes (or steps) _____

Strength Training

GOAL: Sets _____ Repetitions per set _____ Days per week _____

Strength-Training Exercise	Weight/Resistance	Reps	Sets
_____			
_____			
_____			
_____			
_____			
_____			

Stretches

GOAL: Stretches _____ Days per week _____

Stretch	
_____	_____
_____	_____
_____	

Core Exercises

GOAL: Sets _____ Repetitions per set _____ Days per week _____

Core Exercise	Reps	Sets
_____		
_____		
_____		
_____		
_____		
_____		

Additional lifetime/recreational activities? **Y N**

Type: _____

DIET CHECKLIST

Type of Food	Ideal Number of Servings	Breakfast	Lunch	Dinner	Snack(s)	Total Daily Servings
Fruits						
Vegetables (and herbs and spices)						
Grains/legumes/ starchy vegetables						
Milk/yogurt (fat-free or 1%)/soy milk						
High-protein foods						
Nuts/nut butters/seeds						
Healthy fats						
Water						
Superfoods						
Treats/beverages						

Superfoods consumed today (see the list in *20 Years Younger*) _____

_____

Did you take a multivitamin/mineral or other supplement(s)? Y N

SKIN CARE

A.M. Regimen/Products _____

_____

P.M. Regimen/Products _____

_____

Did you apply sunscreen? Y N

SLEEP

GOAL: Hours per night _____

Did you meet this goal today? Y N

WEEK EIGHT   DATE:

Physical Activity

20 YEARS YOUNGER EXERCISE LEVEL: I   II   III

Cardiovascular Exercise

GOAL: Minutes (or steps) per week _____ Today's minutes (or steps) _____

Strength Training

GOAL: Sets _____ Repetitions per set _____ Days per week _____

Strength-Training Exercise	Weight/Resistance	Reps	Sets
_____			
_____			
_____			
_____			
_____			

Stretches

GOAL: Stretches _____ Days per week _____

Stretch

_____   _____

_____   _____

_____

Core Exercises

GOAL: Sets _____ Repetitions per set _____ Days per week _____

Core Exercise	Reps	Sets
_____		
_____		
_____		
_____		
_____		

Additional lifetime/recreational activities? **Y N**

Type: _____

DIET CHECKLIST

Type of Food	Ideal Number of Servings	Breakfast	Lunch	Dinner	Snack(s)	Total Daily Servings
Fruits						
Vegetables (and herbs and spices)						
Grains/legumes/ starchy vegetables						
Milk/yogurt (fat-free or 1%)/soy milk						
High-protein foods						
Nuts/nut butters/seeds						
Healthy fats						
Water						
Superfoods						
Treats/beverages						

Superfoods consumed today (see the list in *20 Years Younger*) _____

_____

Did you take a multivitamin/mineral or other supplement(s)? Y N

SKIN CARE

A.M. Regimen/Products _____

_____

P.M. Regimen/Products _____

_____

Did you apply sunscreen? Y N

SLEEP

GOAL: Hours per night _____

Did you meet this goal today? Y N

WEEKLY SUMMARY

WEEK EIGHT

DATE:

20 YEARS YOUNGER EXERCISE LEVEL: I   II   III

PHYSICAL ACTIVITY

Cardiovascular Exercise

GOAL: Minutes (or steps) per week _____

Did you meet or exceed this goal? Y N

Strength Training

GOAL: Number of exercises _____ Sets _____

Repetitions per set _____ Days per week _____

Did you meet or exceed this goal? Y N

Stretches

GOAL: Stretches _____ Days per week _____

Did you meet or exceed this goal? Y N

Core Exercises

GOAL: Exercises _____ Sets _____

Repetitions per set _____ Days per week _____

Did you meet or exceed this goal? Y N

Lifetime/Recreational Activities

GOAL: Time(s) per week _____

Did you meet or exceed this goal? Y N

DIET

GOAL: Eat the ideal number of servings from each food group —
or get very close — at least five days a week

Did you meet or exceed this goal? Y N

GOAL: Eat at least one superfood from each food group daily

Did you meet or exceed this goal? Y N

GOAL: Take a multivitamin/mineral or other supplement(s) daily

Did you meet this goal? Y N

Skin Care

GOAL: Perform skin care regimen daily in the a.m. and p.m.

Did you meet this goal? Y N

GOAL: Apply sunscreen when needed

Did you meet this goal? Y N

Sleep

GOAL: Hours per night _____

Did you meet this goal? Y N

Notes

_____
_____
_____
_____
_____
_____
_____
_____
_____
_____
_____
_____
_____
_____
_____
_____
_____
_____
_____
_____
_____
_____
_____
_____

WEEK NINE

WEEK NINE DATE: _____

PHYSICAL ACTIVITY

20 YEARS YOUNGER EXERCISE LEVEL: I   II   III

Cardiovascular Exercise

GOAL: Minutes (or steps) per week _____ Today's minutes (or steps) _____

Strength Training

GOAL: Sets _____ Repetitions per set _____ Days per week _____

Strength-Training Exercise	Weight/Resistance	Reps	Sets

Stretches

GOAL: Stretches _____ Days per week _____

Stretch	

Core Exercises

GOAL: Sets _____ Repetitions per set _____ Days per week _____

Core Exercise	Reps	Sets

Additional lifetime/recreational activities? Y N

Type: _____

DIET CHECKLIST

Type of Food	Ideal Number of Servings	Breakfast	Lunch	Dinner	Snack(s)	Total Daily Servings
Fruits						
Vegetables (and herbs and spices)						
Grains/legumes/ starchy vegetables						
Milk/yogurt (fat-free or 1%)/soy milk						
High-protein foods						
Nuts/nut butters/seeds						
Healthy fats						
Water						
Superfoods						
Treats/beverages						

Superfoods consumed today (see the list in *20 Years Younger*) _____

_____

Did you take a multivitamin/mineral or other supplement(s)? Y N

SKIN CARE

A.M. Regimen/Products _____

_____

P.M. Regimen/Products _____

_____

Did you apply sunscreen? Y N

SLEEP

GOAL: Hours per night _____

Did you meet this goal today? Y N

WEEK NINE   DATE:

Physical Activity

20 YEARS YOUNGER EXERCISE LEVEL: I   II   III

Cardiovascular Exercise

GOAL: Minutes (or steps) per week _____ Today's minutes (or steps) _____

Strength Training

GOAL: Sets _____ Repetitions per set _____ Days per week _____

Strength-Training Exercise	Weight/Resistance	Reps	Sets
_____			
_____			
_____			
_____			
_____			
_____			

Stretches

GOAL: Stretches _____ Days per week _____

Stretch

_____	_____
_____	_____
_____	

Core Exercises

GOAL: Sets _____ Repetitions per set _____ Days per week _____

Core Exercise	Reps	Sets
_____		
_____		
_____		
_____		
_____		
_____		

Additional lifetime/recreational activities? **Y N**

Type: _____

DIET CHECKLIST

Type of Food	Ideal Number of Servings	Breakfast	Lunch	Dinner	Snack(s)	Total Daily Servings
Fruits						
Vegetables (and herbs and spices)						
Grains/legumes/ starchy vegetables						
Milk/yogurt (fat-free or 1%)/soy milk						
High-protein foods						
Nuts/nut butters/seeds						
Healthy fats						
Water						
Superfoods						
Treats/beverages						

Superfoods consumed today (see the list in *20 Years Younger*) _____

_____

Did you take a multivitamin/mineral or other supplement(s)? Y N

SKIN CARE

A.M. Regimen/Products _____

_____

P.M. Regimen/Products _____

_____

Did you apply sunscreen? Y N

SLEEP

GOAL: Hours per night _____

Did you meet this goal today? Y N

WEEK NINE   DATE:

Physical Activity

20 YEARS YOUNGER EXERCISE LEVEL: I   II   III

Cardiovascular Exercise

GOAL: Minutes (or steps) per week _____ Today's minutes (or steps) _____

Strength Training

GOAL: Sets _____ Repetitions per set _____ Days per week _____

Strength-Training Exercise	Weight/Resistance	Reps	Sets
_____			
_____			
_____			
_____			
_____			

Stretches

GOAL: Stretches _____ Days per week _____

Stretch	
_____	_____
_____	_____
_____	

Core Exercises

GOAL: Sets _____ Repetitions per set _____ Days per week _____

Core Exercise	Reps	Sets
_____		
_____		
_____		
_____		
_____		

Additional lifetime/recreational activities? **Y N**

Type: _____

DIET CHECKLIST

Type of Food	Ideal Number of Servings	Breakfast	Lunch	Dinner	Snack(s)	Total Daily Servings
Fruits						
Vegetables (and herbs and spices)						
Grains/legumes/ starchy vegetables						
Milk/yogurt (fat-free or 1%)/soy milk						
High-protein foods						
Nuts/nut butters/seeds						
Healthy fats						
Water						
Superfoods						
Treats/beverages						

Superfoods consumed today (see the list in *20 Years Younger*) _____
_____

Did you take a multivitamin/mineral or other supplement(s)? **Y N**

SKIN CARE

A.M. Regimen/Products _____
_____

P.M. Regimen/Products _____
_____

Did you apply sunscreen? **Y N**

SLEEP

GOAL: Hours per night _____

Did you meet this goal today? **Y N**

WEEK NINE   DATE:

Physical Activity

20 YEARS YOUNGER EXERCISE LEVEL: I   II   III

Cardiovascular Exercise

GOAL: Minutes (or steps) per week _____ Today's minutes (or steps) _____

Strength Training

GOAL: Sets _____ Repetitions per set _____ Days per week _____

Strength-Training Exercise	Weight/Resistance	Reps	Sets
_____			
_____			
_____			
_____			
_____			

Stretches

GOAL: Stretches _____ Days per week _____

Stretch	
_____	_____
_____	_____
_____	

Core Exercises

GOAL: Sets _____ Repetitions per set _____ Days per week _____

Core Exercise	Reps	Sets
_____		
_____		
_____		
_____		
_____		

Additional lifetime/recreational activities? Y N

Type: _____

> *The secret to success is constancy of purpose.*
> — BENJAMIN DISRAELI

DIET CHECKLIST

Type of Food	Ideal Number of Servings	Breakfast	Lunch	Dinner	Snack(s)	Total Daily Servings
Fruits						
Vegetables (and herbs and spices)						
Grains/legumes/ starchy vegetables						
Milk/yogurt (fat-free or 1%)/soy milk						
High-protein foods						
Nuts/nut butters/seeds						
Healthy fats						
Water						
Superfoods						
Treats/beverages						

Superfoods consumed today (see the list in *20 Years Younger*) _____

_____

Did you take a multivitamin/mineral or other supplement(s)? Y N

SKIN CARE

A.M. Regimen/Products _____

_____

P.M. Regimen/Products _____

_____

Did you apply sunscreen? Y N

SLEEP

GOAL: Hours per night _____

Did you meet this goal today? Y N

WEEK NINE DATE:

PHYSICAL ACTIVITY

20 YEARS YOUNGER EXERCISE LEVEL: I   II   III

Cardiovascular Exercise

GOAL: Minutes (or steps) per week _____ Today's minutes (or steps) _____

Strength Training

GOAL: Sets _____ Repetitions per set _____ Days per week _____

Strength-Training Exercise	Weight/Resistance	Reps	Sets

Stretches

GOAL: Stretches _____ Days per week _____

Stretch

_____   _____

_____   _____

_____

Core Exercises

GOAL: Sets _____ Repetitions per set _____ Days per week _____

Core Exercise	Reps	Sets

Additional lifetime/recreational activities? **Y N**

Type: _____

DIET CHECKLIST

Type of Food	Ideal Number of Servings	Breakfast	Lunch	Dinner	Snack(s)	Total Daily Servings
Fruits						
Vegetables (and herbs and spices)						
Grains/legumes/ starchy vegetables						
Milk/yogurt (fat-free or 1%)/soy milk						
High-protein foods						
Nuts/nut butters/seeds						
Healthy fats						
Water						
Superfoods						
Treats/beverages						

Superfoods consumed today (see the list in *20 Years Younger*) _____

_____

Did you take a multivitamin/mineral or other supplement(s)? Y N

SKIN CARE

A.M. Regimen/Products _____

_____

P.M. Regimen/Products _____

_____

Did you apply sunscreen? Y N

SLEEP

GOAL: Hours per night _____

Did you meet this goal today? Y N

WEEK NINE   DATE: _____

Physical Activity

20 YEARS YOUNGER EXERCISE LEVEL: I   II   III

Cardiovascular Exercise

GOAL: Minutes (or steps) per week _____ Today's minutes (or steps) _____

Strength Training

GOAL: Sets _____ Repetitions per set _____ Days per week _____

Strength-Training Exercise	Weight/Resistance	Reps	Sets
_____			
_____			
_____			
_____			
_____			
_____			

Stretches

GOAL: Stretches _____ Days per week _____

Stretch

_____   _____

_____   _____

_____

Core Exercises

GOAL: Sets _____ Repetitions per set _____ Days per week _____

Core Exercise	Reps	Sets
_____		
_____		
_____		
_____		
_____		
_____		

Additional lifetime/recreational activities? **Y N**

Type: _____

> *Nothing will work unless you do.*
> — MAYA ANGELOU

DIET CHECKLIST

Type of Food	Ideal Number of Servings	Breakfast	Lunch	Dinner	Snack(s)	Total Daily Servings
Fruits						
Vegetables (and herbs and spices)						
Grains/legumes/ starchy vegetables						
Milk/yogurt (fat-free or 1%)/soy milk						
High-protein foods						
Nuts/nut butters/seeds						
Healthy fats						
Water						
Superfoods						
Treats/beverages						

Superfoods consumed today (see the list in *20 Years Younger*) _____

_____

Did you take a multivitamin/mineral or other supplement(s)? Y N

SKIN CARE

A.M. Regimen/Products _____

_____

P.M. Regimen/Products _____

_____

Did you apply sunscreen? Y N

SLEEP

GOAL: Hours per night _____

Did you meet this goal today? Y N

WEEK NINE   DATE:

Physical Activity

20 YEARS YOUNGER EXERCISE LEVEL: I   II   III

Cardiovascular Exercise

GOAL: Minutes (or steps) per week _____ Today's minutes (or steps) _____

Strength Training

GOAL: Sets _____ Repetitions per set _____ Days per week _____

Strength-Training Exercise	Weight/Resistance	Reps	Sets

Stretches

GOAL: Stretches _____ Days per week _____

Stretch	

Core Exercises

GOAL: Sets _____ Repetitions per set _____ Days per week _____

Core Exercise	Reps	Sets

Additional lifetime/recreational activities? Y N

Type: _____

DIET CHECKLIST

Type of Food	Ideal Number of Servings	Breakfast	Lunch	Dinner	Snack(s)	Total Daily Servings
Fruits						
Vegetables (and herbs and spices)						
Grains/legumes/ starchy vegetables						
Milk/yogurt (fat-free or 1%)/soy milk						
High-protein foods						
Nuts/nut butters/seeds						
Healthy fats						
Water						
Superfoods						
Treats/beverages						

Superfoods consumed today (see the list in *20 Years Younger*) _____

_____

Did you take a multivitamin/mineral or other supplement(s)? Y N

SKIN CARE

A.M. Regimen/Products _____

_____

P.M. Regimen/Products _____

_____

Did you apply sunscreen? Y N

SLEEP

GOAL: Hours per night _____

Did you meet this goal today? Y N

WEEKLY SUMMARY

WEEK NINE   DATE:

PHYSICAL ACTIVITY

Cardiovascular Exercise

GOAL: Minutes (or steps) per week _____

Did you meet or exceed this goal? Y N

Strength Training

GOAL: Number of exercises _____ Sets _____
      Repetitions per set _____ Days per week _____

Did you meet or exceed this goal? Y N

Stretches

GOAL: Stretches _____ Days per week _____

Did you meet or exceed this goal? Y N

Core Exercises

GOAL: Exercises _____ Sets _____
      Repetitions per set _____ Days per week _____

Did you meet or exceed this goal? Y N

Lifetime/Recreational Activities

GOAL: Time(s) per week _____

Did you meet or exceed this goal? Y N

DIET

GOAL: Eat the ideal number of servings from each food group —
      or get very close — at least five days a week

Did you meet or exceed this goal? Y N

GOAL: Eat at least one superfood from each food group daily

Did you meet or exceed this goal? Y N

GOAL: Take a multivitamin/mineral or other supplement(s) daily

Did you meet this goal? Y N

Skin Care

GOAL: Perform skin care regimen daily in the a.m. and p.m.

Did you meet this goal? Y N

GOAL: Apply sunscreen when needed

Did you meet this goal? Y N

Sleep

GOAL: Hours per night _____

Did you meet this goal? Y N

Notes

_____

_____

_____

_____

_____

_____

_____

_____

_____

_____

_____

_____

_____

_____

_____

_____

_____

_____

_____

_____

_____

_____

WEEK TEN

WEEK TEN   DATE:

PHYSICAL ACTIVITY

20 YEARS YOUNGER EXERCISE LEVEL: I II III

Cardiovascular Exercise

GOAL: Minutes (or steps) per week _____ Today's minutes (or steps) _____

Strength Training

GOAL: Sets _____ Repetitions per set _____ Days per week _____

Strength-Training Exercise	Weight/Resistance	Reps	Sets

Stretches

GOAL: Stretches _____ Days per week _____

Stretch	

Core Exercises

GOAL: Sets _____ Repetitions per set _____ Days per week _____

Core Exercise	Reps	Sets

Additional lifetime/recreational activities? Y N

Type: _____

DIET CHECKLIST

Type of Food	Ideal Number of Servings	Breakfast	Lunch	Dinner	Snack(s)	Total Daily Servings
Fruits						
Vegetables (and herbs and spices)						
Grains/legumes/ starchy vegetables						
Milk/yogurt (fat-free or 1%)/soy milk						
High-protein foods						
Nuts/nut butters/seeds						
Healthy fats						
Water						
Superfoods						
Treats/beverages						

Superfoods consumed today (see the list in *20 Years Younger*) _____

_____

Did you take a multivitamin/mineral or other supplement(s)? Y N

SKIN CARE

A.M. Regimen/Products _____

_____

P.M. Regimen/Products _____

_____

Did you apply sunscreen? Y N

SLEEP

GOAL: Hours per night _____

Did you meet this goal today? Y N

WEEK TEN   DATE: _____

PHYSICAL ACTIVITY

20 YEARS YOUNGER EXERCISE LEVEL: I   II   III

Cardiovascular Exercise

GOAL: Minutes (or steps) per week _____ Today's minutes (or steps) _____

Strength Training

GOAL: Sets _____ Repetitions per set _____ Days per week _____

Strength-Training Exercise	Weight/Resistance	Reps	Sets

Stretches

GOAL: Stretches _____ Days per week _____

Stretch	

Core Exercises

GOAL: Sets _____ Repetitions per set _____ Days per week _____

Core Exercise	Reps	Sets

Additional lifetime/recreational activities? Y N

Type: _____

> *It's easier and more enjoyable to do just about any activity when you're in possession of overall fitness.*
>
> — BOB GREENE

DIET CHECKLIST

Type of Food	Ideal Number of Servings	Breakfast	Lunch	Dinner	Snack(s)	Total Daily Servings
Fruits						
Vegetables (and herbs and spices)						
Grains/legumes/ starchy vegetables						
Milk/yogurt (fat-free or 1%)/soy milk						
High-protein foods						
Nuts/nut butters/seeds						
Healthy fats						
Water						
Superfoods						
Treats/beverages						

Superfoods consumed today (see the list in *20 Years Younger*) _____

_____

Did you take a multivitamin/mineral or other supplement(s)? Y N

SKIN CARE

A.M. Regimen/Products _____

_____

P.M. Regimen/Products _____

_____

Did you apply sunscreen? Y N

SLEEP

GOAL: Hours per night _____

Did you meet this goal today? Y N

WEEK TEN   DATE:

Physical Activity

20 YEARS YOUNGER EXERCISE LEVEL: I   II   III

Cardiovascular Exercise

GOAL: Minutes (or steps) per week _____ Today's minutes (or steps) _____

Strength Training

GOAL: Sets _____ Repetitions per set _____ Days per week _____

Strength-Training Exercise	Weight/Resistance	Reps	Sets
_____			
_____			
_____			
_____			
_____			

Stretches

GOAL: Stretches _____ Days per week _____

Stretch	
_____	_____
_____	_____
_____	

Core Exercises

GOAL: Sets _____ Repetitions per set _____ Days per week _____

Core Exercise	Reps	Sets
_____		
_____		
_____		
_____		
_____		
_____		

Additional lifetime/recreational activities? Y N

Type: _____

> *To know how to grow old is the masterwork of wisdom, and one of the most difficult chapters in the great art of living.*
> — HENRI-FRÉDÉRIC AMIEL, *JOURNAL INTIME*

DIET CHECKLIST

Type of Food	Ideal Number of Servings	Breakfast	Lunch	Dinner	Snack(s)	Total Daily Servings
Fruits						
Vegetables (and herbs and spices)						
Grains/legumes/ starchy vegetables						
Milk/yogurt (fat-free or 1%)/soy milk						
High-protein foods						
Nuts/nut butters/seeds						
Healthy fats						
Water						
Superfoods						
Treats/beverages						

Superfoods consumed today (see the list in *20 Years Younger*) _____

_____

Did you take a multivitamin/mineral or other supplement(s)? Y N

SKIN CARE

A.M. Regimen/Products _____

_____

P.M. Regimen/Products _____

_____

Did you apply sunscreen? Y N

SLEEP

GOAL: Hours per night _____

Did you meet this goal today? Y N

WEEK TEN   DATE: _____

Physical Activity

Cardiovascular Exercise

GOAL: Minutes (or steps) per week _____ Today's minutes (or steps) _____

Strength Training

GOAL: Sets _____ Repetitions per set _____ Days per week _____

Strength-Training Exercise	Weight/Resistance	Reps	Sets
_____			
_____			
_____			
_____			
_____			
_____			

Stretches

GOAL: Stretches _____ Days per week _____

Stretch	
_____	_____
_____	_____
_____	

Core Exercises

GOAL: Sets _____ Repetitions per set _____ Days per week _____

Core Exercise	Reps	Sets
_____		
_____		
_____		
_____		
_____		
_____		

Additional lifetime/recreational activities? Y N

Type: _____

> *We don't see things as they are, we see them as we are.*
> — ANAÏS NIN

DIET CHECKLIST

Type of Food	Ideal Number of Servings	Breakfast	Lunch	Dinner	Snack(s)	Total Daily Servings
Fruits						
Vegetables (and herbs and spices)						
Grains/legumes/ starchy vegetables						
Milk/yogurt (fat-free or 1%)/soy milk						
High-protein foods						
Nuts/nut butters/seeds						
Healthy fats						
Water						
Superfoods						
Treats/beverages						

Superfoods consumed today (see the list in *20 Years Younger*) _____

_____

Did you take a multivitamin/mineral or other supplement(s)? Y N

SKIN CARE

A.M. Regimen/Products _____

_____

P.M. Regimen/Products _____

_____

Did you apply sunscreen? Y N

SLEEP

GOAL: Hours per night _____

Did you meet this goal today? Y N

WEEK TEN   DATE: _____

PHYSICAL ACTIVITY

20 YEARS YOUNGER EXERCISE LEVEL: I   II   III

Cardiovascular Exercise

GOAL: Minutes (or steps) per week _____ Today's minutes (or steps) _____

Strength Training

GOAL: Sets _____ Repetitions per set _____ Days per week _____

Strength-Training Exercise	Weight/Resistance	Reps	Sets

Stretches

GOAL: Stretches _____ Days per week _____

Stretch	
_____	_____
_____	_____
_____	

Core Exercises

GOAL: Sets _____ Repetitions per set _____ Days per week _____

Core Exercise	Reps	Sets

Additional lifetime/recreational activities? Y N

Type: _____

DIET CHECKLIST

Type of Food	Ideal Number of Servings	Breakfast	Lunch	Dinner	Snack(s)	Total Daily Servings
Fruits						
Vegetables (and herbs and spices)						
Grains/legumes/ starchy vegetables						
Milk/yogurt (fat-free or 1%)/soy milk						
High-protein foods						
Nuts/nut butters/seeds						
Healthy fats						
Water						
Superfoods						
Treats/beverages						

Superfoods consumed today (see the list in *20 Years Younger*) _____

_____

Did you take a multivitamin/mineral or other supplement(s)? Y N

SKIN CARE

A.M. Regimen/Products _____

_____

P.M. Regimen/Products _____

_____

Did you apply sunscreen? Y N

SLEEP

GOAL: Hours per night _____

Did you meet this goal today? Y N

WEEK TEN   DATE:

Physical Activity

20 YEARS YOUNGER EXERCISE LEVEL: I   II   III

Cardiovascular Exercise

GOAL: Minutes (or steps) per week _____ Today's minutes (or steps) _____

Strength Training

GOAL: Sets _____ Repetitions per set _____ Days per week _____

Strength-Training Exercise	Weight/Resistance	Reps	Sets

Stretches

GOAL: Stretches _____ Days per week _____

Stretch	

Core Exercises

GOAL: Sets _____ Repetitions per set _____ Days per week _____

Core Exercise	Reps	Sets

Additional lifetime/recreational activities? Y N

Type: _____

> *If you think you can do a thing or think you can't do a thing, you're right.*
>
> — HENRY FORD

DIET CHECKLIST

Type of Food	Ideal Number of Servings	Breakfast	Lunch	Dinner	Snack(s)	Total Daily Servings
Fruits						
Vegetables (and herbs and spices)						
Grains/legumes/ starchy vegetables						
Milk/yogurt (fat-free or 1%)/soy milk						
High-protein foods						
Nuts/nut butters/seeds						
Healthy fats						
Water						
Superfoods						
Treats/beverages						

Superfoods consumed today (see the list in *20 Years Younger*) _____

_____

Did you take a multivitamin/mineral or other supplement(s)? Y N

SKIN CARE

A.M. Regimen/Products _____

_____

P.M. Regimen/Products _____

_____

Did you apply sunscreen? Y N

SLEEP

GOAL: Hours per night _____

Did you meet this goal today? Y N

WEEK TEN   DATE:

PHYSICAL ACTIVITY

20 YEARS YOUNGER EXERCISE LEVEL: I   II   III

Cardiovascular Exercise

GOAL: Minutes (or steps) per week _____ Today's minutes (or steps) _____

Strength Training

GOAL: Sets _____ Repetitions per set _____ Days per week _____

Strength-Training Exercise	Weight/Resistance	Reps	Sets

Stretches

GOAL: Stretches _____ Days per week _____

Stretch	

Core Exercises

GOAL: Sets _____ Repetitions per set _____ Days per week _____

Core Exercise	Reps	Sets

Additional lifetime/recreational activities? Y N

Type: _____

> *The will to win, the desire to succeed, the urge to reach your full potential…these are the keys that will unlock the door to personal excellence.*
>
> — CONFUCIUS

DIET CHECKLIST

Type of Food	Ideal Number of Servings	Breakfast	Lunch	Dinner	Snack(s)	Total Daily Servings
Fruits						
Vegetables (and herbs and spices)						
Grains/legumes/ starchy vegetables						
Milk/yogurt (fat-free or 1%)/soy milk						
High-protein foods						
Nuts/nut butters/seeds						
Healthy fats						
Water						
Superfoods						
Treats/beverages						

Superfoods consumed today (see the list in *20 Years Younger*) _____

_____

Did you take a multivitamin/mineral or other supplement(s)? Y N

SKIN CARE

A.M. Regimen/Products _____

_____

P.M. Regimen/Products _____

_____

Did you apply sunscreen? Y N

SLEEP

GOAL: Hours per night _____

Did you meet this goal today? Y N

WEEKLY SUMMARY

WEEK TEN

DATE:

20 YEARS YOUNGER EXERCISE LEVEL: I   II   III

Physical Activity

Cardiovascular Exercise

GOAL: Minutes (or steps) per week _____

Did you meet or exceed this goal? Y N

Strength Training

GOAL: Number of exercises _____ Sets _____

Repetitions per set _____ Days per week _____

Did you meet or exceed this goal? Y N

Stretches

GOAL: Stretches _____ Days per week _____

Did you meet or exceed this goal? Y N

Core Exercises

GOAL: Exercises _____ Sets _____

Repetitions per set _____ Days per week _____

Did you meet or exceed this goal? Y N

Lifetime/Recreational Activities

GOAL: Time(s) per week _____

Did you meet or exceed this goal? Y N

Diet

GOAL: Eat the ideal number of servings from each food group —
or get very close — at least five days a week

Did you meet or exceed this goal? Y N

GOAL: Eat at least one superfood from each food group daily

Did you meet or exceed this goal? Y N

GOAL: Take a multivitamin/mineral or other supplement(s) daily

Did you meet this goal? Y N

Skin Care

GOAL: Perform skin care regimen daily in the a.m. and p.m.

Did you meet this goal? Y N

GOAL: Apply sunscreen when needed

Did you meet this goal? Y N

Sleep

GOAL: Hours per night _____

Did you meet this goal? Y N

Notes

_____
_____
_____
_____
_____
_____
_____
_____
_____
_____
_____
_____
_____
_____
_____
_____
_____
_____
_____
_____
_____
_____
_____
_____

WEEK ELEVEN

WEEK ELEVEN   DATE:

PHYSICAL ACTIVITY

20 YEARS YOUNGER EXERCISE LEVEL: I   II   III

Cardiovascular Exercise

GOAL: Minutes (or steps) per week _____ Today's minutes (or steps) _____

Strength Training

GOAL: Sets _____ Repetitions per set _____ Days per week _____

Strength-Training Exercise	Weight/Resistance	Reps	Sets

Stretches

GOAL: Stretches _____ Days per week _____

Stretch

_____   _____

_____   _____

_____

Core Exercises

GOAL: Sets _____ Repetitions per set _____ Days per week _____

Core Exercise	Reps	Sets

Additional lifetime/recreational activities? Y N

Type: _____

> *How old would you be if you didn't know how old you are?*
> — SATCHEL PAIGE

DIET CHECKLIST

Type of Food	Ideal Number of Servings	Breakfast	Lunch	Dinner	Snack(s)	Total Daily Servings
Fruits						
Vegetables (and herbs and spices)						
Grains/legumes/ starchy vegetables						
Milk/yogurt (fat-free or 1%)/soy milk						
High-protein foods						
Nuts/nut butters/seeds						
Healthy fats						
Water						
Superfoods						
Treats/beverages						

Superfoods consumed today (see the list in *20 Years Younger*) _____

_____

Did you take a multivitamin/mineral or other supplement(s)? Y N

SKIN CARE

A.M. Regimen/Products _____

_____

P.M. Regimen/Products _____

_____

Did you apply sunscreen? Y N

SLEEP

GOAL: Hours per night _____

Did you meet this goal today? Y N

WEEK ELEVEN   DATE: _____

Physical Activity

Cardiovascular Exercise

GOAL: Minutes (or steps) per week _____ Today's minutes (or steps) _____

Strength Training

GOAL: Sets _____ Repetitions per set _____ Days per week _____

Strength-Training Exercise	Weight/Resistance	Reps	Sets

Stretches

GOAL: Stretches _____ Days per week _____

Stretch	

Core Exercises

GOAL: Sets _____ Repetitions per set _____ Days per week _____

Core Exercise	Reps	Sets

Additional lifetime/recreational activities? Y N

Type: _____

> *The only thing that will stop you from fulfilling your dreams is you.*
> — Tom Bradley

Diet Checklist

Type of Food	Ideal Number of Servings	Breakfast	Lunch	Dinner	Snack(s)	Total Daily Servings
Fruits						
Vegetables (and herbs and spices)						
Grains/legumes/ starchy vegetables						
Milk/yogurt (fat-free or 1%)/soy milk						
High-protein foods						
Nuts/nut butters/seeds						
Healthy fats						
Water						
Superfoods						
Treats/beverages						

Superfoods consumed today (see the list in *20 Years Younger*) _____

_____

Did you take a multivitamin/mineral or other supplement(s)? Y N

Skin Care

A.M. Regimen/Products _____

_____

P.M. Regimen/Products _____

_____

Did you apply sunscreen? Y N

Sleep

GOAL: Hours per night _____

Did you meet this goal today? Y N

WEEK ELEVEN   DATE:

Physical Activity

20 YEARS YOUNGER EXERCISE LEVEL: I   II   III

Cardiovascular Exercise

GOAL: Minutes (or steps) per week _____ Today's minutes (or steps) _____

Strength Training

GOAL: Sets _____ Repetitions per set _____ Days per week _____

Strength-Training Exercise	Weight/Resistance	Reps	Sets

Stretches

GOAL: Stretches _____ Days per week _____

Stretch

_____   _____
_____   _____
_____

Core Exercises

GOAL: Sets _____ Repetitions per set _____ Days per week _____

Core Exercise	Reps	Sets

Additional lifetime/recreational activities? Y N

Type: _____

> *Action is the foundational key to all success.*
> — PABLO PICASSO

DIET CHECKLIST

Type of Food	Ideal Number of Servings	Breakfast	Lunch	Dinner	Snack(s)	Total Daily Servings
Fruits						
Vegetables (and herbs and spices)						
Grains/legumes/ starchy vegetables						
Milk/yogurt (fat-free or 1%)/soy milk						
High-protein foods						
Nuts/nut butters/seeds						
Healthy fats						
Water						
Superfoods						
Treats/beverages						

Superfoods consumed today (see the list in *20 Years Younger*) _____

_____

Did you take a multivitamin/mineral or other supplement(s)? **Y N**

SKIN CARE

A.M. Regimen/Products _____

_____

P.M. Regimen/Products _____

_____

Did you apply sunscreen? **Y N**

SLEEP

GOAL: Hours per night _____

Did you meet this goal today? **Y N**

WEEK ELEVEN   DATE:

Physical Activity

Cardiovascular Exercise

GOAL: Minutes (or steps) per week _____ Today's minutes (or steps) _____

Strength Training

GOAL: Sets _____ Repetitions per set _____ Days per week _____

Strength-Training Exercise	Weight/Resistance	Reps	Sets

Stretches

GOAL: Stretches _____ Days per week _____

Stretch

_____   _____
_____   _____
_____

Core Exercises

GOAL: Sets _____ Repetitions per set _____ Days per week _____

Core Exercise	Reps	Sets

Additional lifetime/recreational activities? Y N

Type: _____

> *But if you have nothing at all to create,*
> *then perhaps you create yourself.*
> — CARL JUNG

DIET CHECKLIST

Type of Food	Ideal Number of Servings	Breakfast	Lunch	Dinner	Snack(s)	Total Daily Servings
Fruits						
Vegetables (and herbs and spices)						
Grains/legumes/starchy vegetables						
Milk/yogurt (fat-free or 1%)/soy milk						
High-protein foods						
Nuts/nut butters/seeds						
Healthy fats						
Water						
Superfoods						
Treats/beverages						

Superfoods consumed today (see the list in *20 Years Younger*) _____

_____

Did you take a multivitamin/mineral or other supplement(s)? Y N

SKIN CARE

A.M. Regimen/Products _____

_____

P.M. Regimen/Products _____

_____

Did you apply sunscreen? Y N

SLEEP

GOAL: Hours per night _____
Did you meet this goal today? Y N

WEEK ELEVEN   DATE:

Physical Activity

Cardiovascular Exercise

GOAL: Minutes (or steps) per week _____ Today's minutes (or steps) _____

Strength Training

GOAL: Sets _____ Repetitions per set _____ Days per week _____

Strength-Training Exercise	Weight/Resistance	Reps	Sets

Stretches

GOAL: Stretches _____ Days per week _____

Stretch

_____   _____

_____   _____

_____

Core Exercises

GOAL: Sets _____ Repetitions per set _____ Days per week _____

Core Exercise	Reps	Sets

Additional lifetime/recreational activities? Y N

Type: _____

> *We don't stop playing because we grow old, we grow old because we stop playing.*
>
> — George Bernard Shaw

Diet Checklist

Type of Food	Ideal Number of Servings	Breakfast	Lunch	Dinner	Snack(s)	Total Daily Servings
Fruits						
Vegetables (and herbs and spices)						
Grains/legumes/ starchy vegetables						
Milk/yogurt (fat-free or 1%)/soy milk						
High-protein foods						
Nuts/nut butters/seeds						
Healthy fats						
Water						
Superfoods						
Treats/beverages						

Superfoods consumed today (see the list in *20 Years Younger*) _____

_____

Did you take a multivitamin/mineral or other supplement(s)? **Y N**

Skin Care

A.M. Regimen/Products _____

_____

P.M. Regimen/Products _____

_____

Did you apply sunscreen? **Y N**

Sleep

GOAL: Hours per night _____

Did you meet this goal today? **Y N**

WEEK ELEVEN   DATE:

PHYSICAL ACTIVITY

20 YEARS YOUNGER EXERCISE LEVEL: I   II   III

Cardiovascular Exercise

GOAL: Minutes (or steps) per week _____ Today's minutes (or steps) _____

Strength Training

GOAL: Sets _____ Repetitions per set _____ Days per week _____

Strength-Training Exercise	Weight/Resistance	Reps	Sets

Stretches

GOAL: Stretches _____ Days per week _____

Stretch	

Core Exercises

GOAL: Sets _____ Repetitions per set _____ Days per week _____

Core Exercise	Reps	Sets

Additional lifetime/recreational activities? Y N

Type: _____

> *You cannot expect to achieve new goals or move beyond your present circumstances unless you change.*
> — LES BROWN

DIET CHECKLIST

Type of Food	Ideal Number of Servings	Breakfast	Lunch	Dinner	Snack(s)	Total Daily Servings
Fruits						
Vegetables (and herbs and spices)						
Grains/legumes/ starchy vegetables						
Milk/yogurt (fat-free or 1%)/soy milk						
High-protein foods						
Nuts/nut butters/seeds						
Healthy fats						
Water						
Superfoods						
Treats/beverages						

Superfoods consumed today (see the list in *20 Years Younger*) _____

_____

Did you take a multivitamin/mineral or other supplement(s)? **Y N**

SKIN CARE

A.M. Regimen/Products _____

_____

P.M. Regimen/Products _____

_____

Did you apply sunscreen? **Y N**

SLEEP

GOAL: Hours per night _____

Did you meet this goal today? **Y N**

WEEK ELEVEN   DATE:

Physical Activity

20 YEARS YOUNGER EXERCISE LEVEL: I   II   III

Cardiovascular Exercise

GOAL: Minutes (or steps) per week _____ Today's minutes (or steps) _____

Strength Training

GOAL: Sets _____ Repetitions per set _____ Days per week _____

Strength-Training Exercise	Weight/Resistance	Reps	Sets

Stretches

GOAL: Stretches _____ Days per week _____

Stretch	

Core Exercises

GOAL: Sets _____ Repetitions per set _____ Days per week _____

Core Exercise	Reps	Sets

Additional lifetime/recreational activities? **Y N**

Type: _____

> *There are a lot of keys to happiness;*
> *determine the key to yours.*
> — BOB GREENE

DIET CHECKLIST

Type of Food	Ideal Number of Servings	Breakfast	Lunch	Dinner	Snack(s)	Total Daily Servings
Fruits						
Vegetables (and herbs and spices)						
Grains/legumes/ starchy vegetables						
Milk/yogurt (fat-free or 1%)/soy milk						
High-protein foods						
Nuts/nut butters/seeds						
Healthy fats						
Water						
Superfoods						
Treats/beverages						

Superfoods consumed today (see the list in *20 Years Younger*) _____

Did you take a multivitamin/mineral or other supplement(s)? Y N

SKIN CARE

A.M. Regimen/Products _____

_____

P.M. Regimen/Products _____

_____

Did you apply sunscreen? Y N

SLEEP

GOAL: Hours per night _____

Did you meet this goal today? Y N

WEEKLY SUMMARY

WEEK ELEVEN   DATE:

Physical Activity

Cardiovascular Exercise

GOAL: Minutes (or steps) per week _____

Did you meet or exceed this goal? Y N

Strength Training

GOAL: Number of exercises _____ Sets _____

Repetitions per set _____ Days per week _____

Did you meet or exceed this goal? Y N

Stretches

GOAL: Stretches _____ Days per week _____

Did you meet or exceed this goal? Y N

Core Exercises

GOAL: Exercises _____ Sets _____

Repetitions per set _____ Days per week _____

Did you meet or exceed this goal? Y N

Lifetime/Recreational Activities

GOAL: Time(s) per week _____

Did you meet or exceed this goal? Y N

Diet

GOAL: Eat the ideal number of servings from each food group —
or get very close — at least five days a week

Did you meet or exceed this goal? Y N

GOAL: Eat at least one superfood from each food group daily

Did you meet or exceed this goal? Y N

GOAL: Take a multivitamin/mineral or other supplement(s) daily

Did you meet this goal? Y N

Skin Care

GOAL: Perform skin care regimen daily in the a.m. and p.m.

Did you meet this goal? Y N

GOAL: Apply sunscreen when needed

Did you meet this goal? Y N

Sleep

GOAL: Hours per night _____

Did you meet this goal? Y N

Notes

_____
_____
_____
_____
_____
_____
_____
_____
_____
_____
_____
_____
_____
_____
_____
_____
_____
_____
_____
_____
_____
_____

WEEK TWELVE

WEEK TWELVE   DATE:

Physical Activity

20 YEARS YOUNGER EXERCISE LEVEL: I   II   III

Cardiovascular Exercise

GOAL: Minutes (or steps) per week _____ Today's minutes (or steps) _____

Strength Training

GOAL: Sets _____ Repetitions per set _____ Days per week _____

Strength-Training Exercise	Weight/Resistance	Reps	Sets

Stretches

GOAL: Stretches _____ Days per week _____

Stretch

_____   _____

_____   _____

_____

Core Exercises

GOAL: Sets _____ Repetitions per set _____ Days per week _____

Core Exercise	Reps	Sets

Additional lifetime/recreational activities? Y N

Type: _____

> *We change our lives. We can do, have,*
> *and be exactly what we wish.*
> — ANTHONY ROBBINS

DIET CHECKLIST

Type of Food	Ideal Number of Servings	Breakfast	Lunch	Dinner	Snack(s)	Total Daily Servings
Fruits						
Vegetables (and herbs and spices)						
Grains/legumes/ starchy vegetables						
Milk/yogurt (fat-free or 1%)/soy milk						
High-protein foods						
Nuts/nut butters/seeds						
Healthy fats						
Water						
Superfoods						
Treats/beverages						

Superfoods consumed today (see the list in *20 Years Younger*) _____

_____

Did you take a multivitamin/mineral or other supplement(s)? Y N

SKIN CARE

A.M. Regimen/Products _____

_____

P.M. Regimen/Products _____

_____

Did you apply sunscreen? Y N

SLEEP

GOAL: Hours per night _____

Did you meet this goal today? Y N

WEEK TWELVE   DATE:

Physical Activity

20 YEARS YOUNGER EXERCISE LEVEL: I   II   III

Cardiovascular Exercise

GOAL: Minutes (or steps) per week _____ Today's minutes (or steps) _____

Strength Training

GOAL: Sets _____ Repetitions per set _____ Days per week _____

Strength-Training Exercise	Weight/Resistance	Reps	Sets

Stretches

GOAL: Stretches _____ Days per week _____

Stretch

Core Exercises

GOAL: Sets _____ Repetitions per set _____ Days per week _____

Core Exercise	Reps	Sets

Additional lifetime/recreational activities? Y N

Type: _____

> *Never neglect an opportunity for improvement.*
> — SIR WILLIAM JONES

DIET CHECKLIST

Type of Food	Ideal Number of Servings	Breakfast	Lunch	Dinner	Snack(s)	Total Daily Servings
Fruits						
Vegetables (and herbs and spices)						
Grains/legumes/ starchy vegetables						
Milk/yogurt (fat-free or 1%)/soy milk						
High-protein foods						
Nuts/nut butters/seeds						
Healthy fats						
Water						
Superfoods						
Treats/beverages						

Superfoods consumed today (see the list in *20 Years Younger*) _____

_____

Did you take a multivitamin/mineral or other supplement(s)? Y N

SKIN CARE

A.M. Regimen/Products _____

_____

P.M. Regimen/Products _____

_____

Did you apply sunscreen? Y N

SLEEP

GOAL: Hours per night _____

Did you meet this goal today? Y N

WEEK TWELVE   DATE:

Physical Activity

20 YEARS YOUNGER EXERCISE LEVEL: I   II   III

Cardiovascular Exercise

GOAL: Minutes (or steps) per week _____ Today's minutes (or steps) _____

Strength Training

GOAL: Sets _____ Repetitions per set _____ Days per week _____

Strength-Training Exercise	Weight/Resistance	Reps	Sets

Stretches

GOAL: Stretches _____ Days per week _____

Stretch	

Core Exercises

GOAL: Sets _____ Repetitions per set _____ Days per week _____

Core Exercise	Reps	Sets

Additional lifetime/recreational activities? Y N

Type: _____

> *Happiness is the real sense of fulfillment that comes from hard work.*
>
> — JOSEPH BARBARA

DIET CHECKLIST

Type of Food	Ideal Number of Servings	Breakfast	Lunch	Dinner	Snack(s)	Total Daily Servings
Fruits						
Vegetables (and herbs and spices)						
Grains/legumes/ starchy vegetables						
Milk/yogurt (fat-free or 1%)/soy milk						
High-protein foods						
Nuts/nut butters/seeds						
Healthy fats						
Water						
Superfoods						
Treats/beverages						

Superfoods consumed today (see the list in *20 Years Younger*) _____

Did you take a multivitamin/mineral or other supplement(s)? Y N

SKIN CARE

A.M. Regimen/Products _____

_____

P.M. Regimen/Products _____

_____

Did you apply sunscreen? Y N

SLEEP

GOAL: Hours per night _____

Did you meet this goal today? Y N

WEEK TWELVE   DATE:

Physical Activity

Cardiovascular Exercise

GOAL: Minutes (or steps) per week _____ Today's minutes (or steps) _____

Strength Training

GOAL: Sets _____ Repetitions per set _____ Days per week _____

Strength-Training Exercise	Weight/Resistance	Reps	Sets

Stretches

GOAL: Stretches _____ Days per week _____

Stretch	

Core Exercises

GOAL: Sets _____ Repetitions per set _____ Days per week _____

Core Exercise	Reps	Sets

Additional lifetime/recreational activities? Y N

Type: _____

> *Nobody can go back and start a new beginning, but anyone can start today and make a new ending.*
> — MARIA ROBINSON

DIET CHECKLIST

Type of Food	Ideal Number of Servings	Breakfast	Lunch	Dinner	Snack(s)	Total Daily Servings
Fruits						
Vegetables (and herbs and spices)						
Grains/legumes/ starchy vegetables						
Milk/yogurt (fat-free or 1%)/soy milk						
High-protein foods						
Nuts/nut butters/seeds						
Healthy fats						
Water						
Superfoods						
Treats/beverages						

Superfoods consumed today (see the list in *20 Years Younger*) _____

_____

Did you take a multivitamin/mineral or other supplement(s)? Y N

SKIN CARE

A.M. Regimen/Products _____

_____

P.M. Regimen/Products _____

_____

Did you apply sunscreen? Y N

SLEEP

GOAL: Hours per night _____

Did you meet this goal today? Y N

WEEK TWELVE   DATE:

PHYSICAL ACTIVITY

20 YEARS YOUNGER EXERCISE LEVEL: I   II   III

Cardiovascular Exercise

GOAL: Minutes (or steps) per week _____ Today's minutes (or steps) _____

Strength Training

GOAL: Sets _____ Repetitions per set _____ Days per week _____

Strength-Training Exercise	Weight/Resistance	Reps	Sets

Stretches

GOAL: Stretches _____ Days per week _____

Stretch

_____   _____

_____   _____

_____

Core Exercises

GOAL: Sets _____ Repetitions per set _____ Days per week _____

Core Exercise	Reps	Sets

Additional lifetime/recreational activities? Y N

Type: _____

DIET CHECKLIST

Type of Food	Ideal Number of Servings	Breakfast	Lunch	Dinner	Snack(s)	Total Daily Servings
Fruits						
Vegetables (and herbs and spices)						
Grains/legumes/ starchy vegetables						
Milk/yogurt (fat-free or 1%)/soy milk						
High-protein foods						
Nuts/nut butters/seeds						
Healthy fats						
Water						
Superfoods						
Treats/beverages						

Superfoods consumed today (see the list in *20 Years Younger*) _____

_____

Did you take a multivitamin/mineral or other supplement(s)? Y N

SKIN CARE

A.M. Regimen/Products _____

_____

P.M. Regimen/Products _____

_____

Did you apply sunscreen? Y N

SLEEP

GOAL: Hours per night _____

Did you meet this goal today? Y N

WEEK TWELVE   DATE:

Physical Activity

20 YEARS YOUNGER EXERCISE LEVEL: I   II   III

Cardiovascular Exercise

GOAL: Minutes (or steps) per week _____ Today's minutes (or steps) _____

Strength Training

GOAL: Sets _____ Repetitions per set _____ Days per week _____

Strength-Training Exercise	Weight/Resistance	Reps	Sets

Stretches

GOAL: Stretches _____ Days per week _____

Stretch	
_____	_____
_____	_____
_____	

Core Exercises

GOAL: Sets _____ Repetitions per set _____ Days per week _____

Core Exercise	Reps	Sets

Additional lifetime/recreational activities? Y N

Type: _____

> *To remain young while growing old is the highest blessing.*
> — GERMAN PROVERB

DIET CHECKLIST

Type of Food	Ideal Number of Servings	Breakfast	Lunch	Dinner	Snack(s)	Total Daily Servings
Fruits						
Vegetables (and herbs and spices)						
Grains/legumes/ starchy vegetables						
Milk/yogurt (fat-free or 1%)/soy milk						
High-protein foods						
Nuts/nut butters/seeds						
Healthy fats						
Water						
Superfoods						
Treats/beverages						

Superfoods consumed today (see the list in *20 Years Younger*) _____

Did you take a multivitamin/mineral or other supplement(s)? Y N

SKIN CARE

A.M. Regimen/Products _____

_____

P.M. Regimen/Products _____

_____

Did you apply sunscreen? Y N

SLEEP

GOAL: Hours per night _____

Did you meet this goal today? Y N

WEEK TWELVE   DATE:

Physical Activity

20 YEARS YOUNGER EXERCISE LEVEL: I   II   III

Cardiovascular Exercise

GOAL: Minutes (or steps) per week _____ Today's minutes (or steps) _____

Strength Training

GOAL: Sets _____ Repetitions per set _____ Days per week _____

Strength-Training Exercise	Weight/Resistance	Reps	Sets

Stretches

GOAL: Stretches _____ Days per week _____

Stretch	

Core Exercises

GOAL: Sets _____ Repetitions per set _____ Days per week _____

Core Exercise	Reps	Sets

Additional lifetime/recreational activities? Y N

Type: _____

> *It is good to have an end to journey towards; but it is the journey that matters in the end.*
> — Ursula K. LeGuin

DIET CHECKLIST

Type of Food	Ideal Number of Servings	Breakfast	Lunch	Dinner	Snack(s)	Total Daily Servings
Fruits						
Vegetables (and herbs and spices)						
Grains/legumes/ starchy vegetables						
Milk/yogurt (fat-free or 1%)/soy milk						
High-protein foods						
Nuts/nut butters/seeds						
Healthy fats						
Water						
Superfoods						
Treats/beverages						

Superfoods consumed today (see the list in *20 Years Younger*) _____

_____

Did you take a multivitamin/mineral or other supplement(s)? Y N

SKIN CARE

A.M. Regimen/Products _____

_____

P.M. Regimen/Products _____

_____

Did you apply sunscreen? Y N

SLEEP

GOAL: Hours per night _____

Did you meet this goal today? Y N

WEEKLY SUMMARY

WEEK TWELVE   DATE:

20 YEARS YOUNGER EXERCISE LEVEL: I   II   III

PHYSICAL ACTIVITY

Cardiovascular Exercise

GOAL: Minutes (or steps) per week _____

Did you meet or exceed this goal? Y N

Strength Training

GOAL: Number of exercises _____ Sets _____

Repetitions per set _____ Days per week _____

Did you meet or exceed this goal? Y N

Stretches

GOAL: Stretches _____ Days per week _____

Did you meet or exceed this goal? Y N

Core Exercises

GOAL: Exercises _____ Sets _____

Repetitions per set _____ Days per week _____

Did you meet or exceed this goal? Y N

Lifetime/Recreational Activities

GOAL: Time(s) per week _____

Did you meet or exceed this goal? Y N

DIET

GOAL: Eat the ideal number of servings from each food group —
or get very close — at least five days a week

Did you meet or exceed this goal? Y N

GOAL: Eat at least one superfood from each food group daily

Did you meet or exceed this goal? Y N

GOAL: Take a multivitamin/mineral or other supplement(s) daily

Did you meet this goal? Y N

Skin Care

GOAL: Perform skin care regimen daily in the a.m. and p.m.

Did you meet this goal? Y N

GOAL: Apply sunscreen when needed

Did you meet this goal? Y N

Sleep

GOAL: Hours per night _____

Did you meet this goal? Y N

Notes

_____

_____

_____

_____

_____

_____

_____

_____

_____

_____

_____

_____

_____

_____

_____

_____

_____

_____

_____

_____

_____

_____

_____

_____

_____